FERTILITY AND HOUSEHOLD LABOUR IN TANZANIA

Fertility and Household Labour in Tanzania

Demography, Economy, and Society in Rufiji District, *c*.1870–1986

Matthew Lockwood

CLARENDON PRESS • OXFORD
1998

This book has been printed digitally and produced in a standard design in order to ensure its continuing availability

OXFORD
UNIVERSITY PRESS

Great Clarendon Street, Oxford OX2 6DP

Oxford University Press is a department of the University of Oxford.
It furthers the University's objective of excellence in research, scholarship,
and education by publishing worldwide in

Oxford New York

Athens Auckland Bangkok Bogotá Buenos Aires Cape Town
Chennai Dar es Salaam Delhi Florence Hong Kong Istanbul Karachi
Kolkata Kuala Lumpur Madrid Melbourne Mexico City Mumbai Nairobi
Paris São Paulo Shanghai Singapore Taipei Tokyo Toronto Warsaw

with associated companies in Berlin Ibadan

Oxford is a registered trade mark of Oxford University Press
in the UK and in certain other countries

Published in the United States
by Oxford University Press Inc., New York

Reprinted 2001

ISBN 0-19-828754-2

Acknowledgements

This book has been a long time in the making. On many occasions the help and support of other people has been crucial. Of course, without the hospitality, insights, and patience of the people of Rufiji, the book would not exist at all. For sharing their home with me in Mng'aru, I would particularly like to thank Jumandera Mtandika, Asala, and Mama Asala. I learned a huge proportion of what little I know about Mng'aru from Moshi Mohammedi Mokea, who was my guide, teacher, and interpreter. I am also grateful to Nyamatimbwa Sultani for her interviewing work. In other parts of the District I enjoyed the hospitality and support of Seif Suleman and his family, and the Norad project staff, especialy Bo Klit Christiansen.

I would also like to thank the friends and colleagues in Dar es Salaam who gave me succor between bouts of fieldwork: Ian Mamuya, Werner Biermann and Gero Erhart, Salim Wanambusi Busolo, John and Rosemarie Campbell, P. P. Namfua, and Marion Kessy. Chrysanth Kamuzora was a guiding and helpful presence.

Most of the book is based on a D. Phil thesis submitted to Oxford University. For the doctorate I was very fortunate to have the sympathetic, incisive, and inspiring supervision of Megan Vaughan, plus the fertile mind of Richard Smith to draw upon. In the process of changing a thesis into a book, I have received encouragement and help from John Iliffe, Pat Caplan, and Ann Whitehead. I am also grateful to the staff of the African Studies Centre, Cambridge University, during the period 1990 to 1992, for their assistance. The demographic sections of the book, especially Chapter 1, have benefited from the extensive comments of an anonymous reader, to whom I am grateful, and also from data from the 1988 Census of Tanzania, generously supplied by Akim Mturi.

For putting up with me while wrestling with the thesis, I am truly indebted to my friends in Oxford and London in the 1980s: Andrew Kilmister, Val Wilson, Jon Lunn, Suzan Quilliam, Jeremy Krikler, Patricia Daley, Tom Forrest, Ena Aracil, Tom Buchanan, Julia Lowndes, Simon Davison, and Helen Napper. For helping me to keep the book in perspective, grateful thanks to Kishti Sheather, and to Alice Myers, who was a constant inspiration.

Finally I would like to acknowledge my debt to my parents; they were generous with their love and financial support. This book is dedicated to them.

Contents

List of Figures viii
List of Maps ix
List of Tables x
Abbreviations xiii
Introduction 1

PART I

Introduction to Part I 11

1. The Historical Demography of Coastal Tanzania **23**
Appendix 1.1: Population of Rufiji District, 1913–86 42

2. The Proximate Determinants of Fertility **44**
Appendix 2.1: Calculation of the Bongaarts and Potter Indices 56

3. The Historical Roots of a Fertility Regime **58**

4. Twentieth-century Transformations **69**

5. Interpretations of Change **86**

PART II

Introduction to Part II 101

6. Labour and Land in Mng'aru **117**

7. Inequality and Accumulation in Mng'aru **132**

8. Households and Life Cycles in Mng'aru: Norms and Patterns **142**

9. Household Demography and Patterns of Work **163**

Conclusion 183
References 187
Index 201

List of Figures

1.1	Child mortality: Coast Region	34
1.2	Child mortality: Rufiji District	35
1.3	Parity progression ratios: Coast Region	38
1.4	Synthetic parity progression ratios: Coast Region, 1988	40
6.1	Seasonal cycles in Mng'aru	119
7.1	Per adult land distribution	133
7.2	Distribution of male tree-crop ownership	134
7.3	Distribution of per capita wealth	137
8.1	C–W differences by life-cycle stage	154
8.2	Life-course paths for women aged 35 and over	158
9.1	Women's rice-growing and children's ages	177

List of Maps

1 Location of Rufiji District 20
2 Rufiji District: villages and roads 110

List of Tables

1.1	The population of Rufiji Disctrict, 1913–1988	29
1.2	The population of Rufiji District, 1913–1988 (selected estimates)	29
1.3	Sex ratios, Rufiji District, 1921–1988	31
1.4	Place of birth of Dar es Salaam residents, 1952–1977	32
1.5	Infant mortality rates, 1913–1991/2	33
1.6	Period total fertility rates, 1948–1991/2	36
1.7	Mean children ever born, Coast Region/Eastern Province	36
1.8	Percentage of women with 0 and 1–2 births, Coast Region/Eastern Province	40
A1.1	Unadjusted estimates of the population of Rufiji District, 1913–1988	42
A1.2	Adjusted estimates of the population of Rufiji District, 1913–1988	43
2.1	Percentage of women married, by age group, Coast Region 1967–1978	53
2.2	Singulate mean ages at marriage, 1973 and 1978, Coast Region	53
2.3	Proximate fertility determination, Rufiji District/Coast Region, 1967–1988	54
4.1	Acreage, harvest, and sales of rice and cotton, Rufiji District, 1925–1937	82
4.2	Purchases of cashews, 1961/2–1981/2	83
4.3	Indices of rural living standards, Tanzania, 1969–1982/3	85
5.1	Polygyny in Coast Region/Eastern Province, 1957–1978	97
6.1	Crops grown in Mng'aru	118
6.2	Normative divisions of labour by gender (adults)	121
6.3	Time spent on tasks by sex (adults aged 16+)	123
6.4	Frequency of tasks performed with or for another (adults)	126
6.5	Frequency of tasks performed with or for another (children)	126
7.1	Plot size distribution	133
7.2	Distribution of tree ownership by age group	135
7.3	Distribution of tree ownership by ex-migrant status	135
7.4	Cashew and wealth ownership, by age of household head	138

7.5 Previous migration and roofing source 138
7.6 Education of household head and asset ownership 138
7.7 Rice-growing, household composition, and wealth 139
7.8 Wealth per adult and men's labour allocation 140
8.1 Variation in number of children by age of household head 150
8.2 Marital status of household heads by age of household head 151
8.3 Sex of household head by age of household head 151
8.4 Variation in household structure by age of household head 152
8.5 Variation in household extension by age of household head 152
8.6 Distribution of households by type: Char Gopalpur and Mng'aru 153
8.7 Primary and secondary sterility (married women) 156
8.8 Parity and surviving children for women aged 35 and over, Mng'aru 156
8.9 Mean number of marriages per woman 157
8.10 Percentage distribution of women by number of marriages, Ikwiriri and Mng'aru 157
8.11 Number of children ever born by number of marriages, women aged 35+, Mng'aru 158
8.12 Wealth and polygyny 159
8.13 Wealth and household extension 160
8.14 Net consumer–worker differences for extended households: nuclear and extended components 161
8.15 Sex composition of extended households: nuclear and extended components 161
9.1 Household size and household participation in secondary activities 166
9.2 Household size and rice-growing 167
9.3 Per adult labour allocation and household size 167
9.4 Mean acreage of land farmed, by number of adults 167
9.5 Per adult labour allocation and consumer-worker differences 168
9.6 Male labour allocation and consumer–worker differences 169
9.7 Female labour allocation and consumer–worker differences 169
9.8 Household type and household participation in secondary activities 171
9.9 Household sex composition and rice cultivation 171

9.10 Women's age and rice-growing 173
9.11 Women's marital status and rice-growing 173
9.12 Women's labour allocation and marital status 174
9.13 Number of young children and women's time-use 175
9.14 Women's time-use by presence of young children and presence of teenage girls 175
9.15 Amount of time spent in domestic work by adult women with young children and with and without teenage girls 176
9.16 Women's rice-gowing and young children in the household 176
9.17 Number of women in the household and women's time-use 177
9.18 Women's rice-growing and number of women in household 178
9.19 Number of men in the household and women's time-use 178
9.20 Men's labour allocation and marital status 179
9.21 Number of other men in the household and men's time-use 179

Abbreviations

BRALUP	Bureau of Resource Assessment and Land-Use Planning, University of Dar es Salaam
CDR	Child death rate
DHS	Demographic and Health Survey
DSM	Dar es Salaam
GLM	General linear models
IMR	Infant mortality rate
IRA	Institute of Resource Assessment, University of Dar es Salaam
MCEB	Mean children ever born
MCH	Maternal and child health
NUMEIST	National Urban Nobility, Employment, and Income Survey of Tanzania
PPR	Parity progression ratio
RH	Rhodes House
RPI	Retail Price Index
SMAM	Singulate mean age at marriage
TANU	Tanganyika African National Union
TDHS	Tanzanian Demographic and Health Survey
TFR	Total fertility rate
TNA	Tanzania National Archives
UMATI	Tanzanian Family-planning Association

Introduction

This book is a study of human, social, and economic reproduction in Rufiji, a district of coastal Tanzania. It contains two parts, each of which addresses a particular question. In the first half I ask how fertility in Rufiji changed over the twentieth century, and what social and economic transformations were involved. In the second half, attention shifts to one village, Mng'aru, and I examine the influence of household demography on the work patterns of men and women.

A guiding theme through the book is a particular approach to the study of reproduction. In this sense, although also an historical and sociological description of Rufiji, the work is at another level an attempt to develop and apply a set of methods for analysing reproduction. Particular notions of reproduction are central to the treatment of history and economy here.

Defining Reproduction

What, then, is 'reproduction'? The term is often used as synonymous for the biological processes of birth and death. However, it can and has also been used to refer to a much wider range of processes—indeed any process involving renewal.

My original impulse to investigate human reproduction did not come through demography, but rather through a desire to understand the day-to-day burdens of domestic work for women in rural Africa, and to locate that understanding within the wider structures of national and world economies. Among the factors influencing the situation of rural African women, child-bearing and rearing appeared to loom large. Furthermore, explanations of high fertility seemed to be tied up with a multitude of other social phenomena and structures: modernization, colonial exploitation, women's education, women's status, the control of men over women, and the exchange of the latter between corporate kin groups, the labour and security value of children.

One writer who paid particular attention to the articulation of domestic relations in Africa, including fertility and marriage, with wider economic structures, was Claude Meillassoux (1981, 1983). Merging Marxist concerns of exchange, production and exploitation with Lévi-Strauss's analysis of kinship, Meillassoux developed the notion of the 'domestic community', in which the labour of junior men and the reproductive powers of women were controlled and exchanged by senior men. Colonial capitalism entered, but did not destroy, the domestic community, producing new strains and greater levels of exploitation.

A distinctive characteristic of Meillassoux's analysis is that it gives central place to the concept of reproduction. For the senior men, the reproduction of the community over time is the objective to be secured. Seeds, tools, and labour are the necessary means of securing this reproduction. The control of women's power to reproduce labour therefore becomes crucial to the reproduction of the community.

Meillassoux produced a powerful framework which focused much-needed attention on the reproduction of labour power in economies. However, his work has been much criticized by feminists, largely because having argued that the subordination of women is 'required' within the domestic community he gives no account of how this might be maintained, or how insubordination might be dealt with (Moore 1988: 49–54). Related to this, there was also a problem with the way in which Meillassoux used the concept of reproduction. Edholm *et al.* (1977) pointed out that there are several distinct meanings or levels of the concept, which become merged together in Meillassoux. This has important implications for the analysis of fertility: 'It is assumed that biological reproduction is merely one, unproblematic, aspect of reproduction as a whole. Human reproduction is analysed as a fundamental part of total social reproduction and analysed within the same conceptual framework' (Edholm *et al.* 1977: 103).

To avoid this error, they suggested a threefold distinction between human (or biological) reproduction, the reproduction of labour, and social reproduction. This last refers to 'the overall reproduction of a particular social formation' (Harris and Young 1981: 113)—specifically the structures and relationships between individuals which 'have to be reproduced in order that social reproduction as a whole can take place' (Edholm *et al.* 1977: 105). Benería specifies social reproduction further by pointing out that it implies the 'transmission of control of resources from one generation to the next'. This includes property, but it can also encompass access to education, to skills, and to power (Benería 1979: 206). As such, its institutions include those of class, race, nation, lineage, family, and marriage.

The reproduction of labour, meanwhile, is distinct, for although 'the reproduction of adequately socialised, adequately nourished labour is a condition of existence for the reproduction of any social system', the forms of allocation, socialization, and daily maintenance of labour do not follow uniformly from the nature of the social system (Harris and Young 1981: 123–4). Edholm *et al.* note a distinction between the daily maintenance of a labour force 'in the here and now', and the allocation of people to positions within the labour process over time. This is to state an important but often neglected fact; the labour force is socially constituted, and the rules of who is a potential worker in a particular process can change over time. Thus an essential element of the reproduction of the labour force is how individuals are allocated to it. Lastly, we have human or biological reproduction, the material conditions of which have changed significantly only recently.

As stated by Edholm *et al.*, their purpose is to avoid conflating all aspects of reproduction into one, and thus the reductionism of their principal target—Meillassoux. Specifically:

> [W]hile clearly the production of human beings, biological reproduction, is a necessary condition for the continued reproduction of the social formation, rates of fertility and the specific conditions of human reproduction cannot be simply derived from, or seen as being in functional harmony with, social reproduction as a whole. (Harris and Young 1981: 113)

This criticism of Meillassoux turns out to be applicable to an extraordinarily wide range of explanations of fertility, from new household economics models, to Caldwell's wealth flows account, to Marxist approaches to African historical demography,[1] to more recent 'cultural' explanations of high fertility in Africa. All of them, in different ways, start with an account of an economic or social system, and move to an explanation of fertility behaviour in terms of its contribution to the maintenance of that system.

It seemed to me that such an explanatory form could also be found in a different kind of analysis of reproduction—that relating the household life cycle to economic mobility in peasant economies. Views tended to polarize into two camps, again based on an initial account of the economic system. If peasant economic relations were seen through a Leninist or neoclassical lens, then household demography was swamped by considerations of capital and labour markets. If a Chayanovian view of the rural economy was taken, the household life cycle determined economic mobility.

When I started the research on which this book is based, I was working within one of these paradigms, namely neoclassical economics. Partly through fieldwork experience (see below), I became dissatisfied with this approach, and, more generally, with the form of explanation described above. I wanted to find a new approach to studying both fertility and the effects of household demography which did not impose systemic assumptions on explanation.

The key move towards this approach came in thinking about explanations of fertility. My analysis of the effects of household demography followed on from this, and is taken up again in the introduction to Part II. My approach to fertility explanation was much influenced by the analysis of proximate determinants, a framework which became available from 1983. This made it possible to start, not with an economic and social system, but first with fertility patterns themselves, and then their proximate determinants, which in turn act as valuable 'pointers' to which social and economic factors may be at work. It is still, of course, possible to introduce functional and systemic accounts even at this point, but the more specific information given by decomposing fertility into its proximate determinants makes it more difficult to sustain explanations which try to impose system on history (see Smith (1981) for a key example).

One of the most important insights to be gained from focusing on the proximate determinants is the significance of modern contraception as a pointer to conscious individual fertility control. As Ansley Coale (1973) has pointed out, this requires not only material motivation, information, and availability, but

[1] For a critique of work by Cordell *et al.* based on the Edholm *et al.* analysis, see Vock (1988).

also a particular way of thinking about one's fertility—that it can and should be controlled directly. The use of modern contraception and the closely related phenomenon of conscious choice are crucial watersheds for the applicability of certain kinds of fertility explanation. For instance, theories based on the notion of an individual- or couple-level 'demand' for children (as with neoclassical economics) are plausible only for societies where people have crossed the watershed of conscious choice. In other cases, fertility determination and change will work through other mechanisms, such as marriage, or a changing period of breastfeeding, which may have little to do with the state of fertility 'preferences'. Thus there are two distinct problems in explanations of fertility. One is how changing fertility relates to economic, social, and cultural change in non-contracepting societies; the second is how non-contracepting societies enter the phase of conscious choice.

Shauri la Mungu—up to God

A recognition of the importance of the proximate determinants of fertility came about only because my fieldwork experience convinced me that the neoclassical approach I had been following was not appropriate for my Tanzanian case. Between August 1985 and November 1986 I lived in Tanzania, for most of that time in Rufiji, in one small village. When I arrived in Tanzania I wanted to study the effects of rural–urban migration on fertility decisions, and had some background material on the floodplain of Rufiji which is near, but not too near, to Dar es Salaam. I quickly found a suitable research site in Mng'aru, which was near to the tarmac road and small enough to enumerate.[2]

Although I thus stuck to my original plans for a research location, my approach to the study of fertility soon began to change as, in the course of living in Mng'aru and observing the parameters within which people lived, increasing tension arose between the economic models of fertility I had brought with me and the way that people thought about fertility.

Neoclassical economics looks at fertility behaviour as if it were the outcome of an economic decision. Other approaches, including Caldwell's wealth-flows model, also emphasize the significance of economic benefits and costs of children to parents. This position has come under increasing attack, on both theoretical and empirical grounds, and the debate still rages without resolution (e.g. Cleland 1993; Thomas 1991, 1993). This is examined in the Introduction to Part I. However, my view of how economic metaphors of fertility behaviour can mislead *in certain cases* came about in the course of fieldwork, in the way that people in Rufiji think about children.

In the 1970s, when empirical research on fertility and the roles of children in Africa was getting under way, much was made of expressions of the economic value of children. It was equally possible to find common expressions of the

[2] It also had a good selection of mango, papaya, and citrus trees, a crucial factor for the fruit-loving fieldworker.

value of children in Mng'aru: 'My wealth (*mali*) is in my children'; 'Children are savings (*akiba*)'; 'Children are important—"children" is an important word'; 'Children are like money—if you have good luck they will help you'; 'When they [children] are grown up and when you are old, they help you.'

However, these identifications of children with wealth, savings, and security in later life were not the only things that people had to say about children. Just as frequent were the qualifications that this all depended on the relationship between parent and child; on the character and *akili*, or skill and intelligence of the child; and on good luck (*bahati*). Returns to having children then, like many other activities, are hedged round with great uncertainty:

If children are still small you don't get any profit at all, but when they are grown up they might help you. It depends on the nature of the child, and on their *akili*.

When children move [to the city], some help their parents and some don't; some send their parents money and gifts regularly, others just forget them and spend their money on clothes and dancing.

If you are in hospital, they come for one day and just leave fifty shillings because they want to get back to the life of the city. There are many like that.

If you are lucky, you will be helped if you have children. But it depends on the character (*asili*) of the child—some, even if they get to school or college, just drink beer and smoke marijuana, and are thrown out.

Parents, and indeed adults generally, have a realistic view of children: they are an important form of security and income in later years, in the absence of other sources of these things, but not a certain one. They can also be a costly burden to raise. You cannot necessarily control children, and, as Terence Hull puts it, each child brings its own fortune. The result is a pronatalist society, but one in which the idea of controlling fertility in response to the economic value of children is still alien.

In informal conversation with villagers about children, they would usually reply to my questions about how many they wanted by saying '*Ni shauri la Mungu*' which roughly translates as the 'Up to God' response familiar to demographers. In the World Fertility Surveys held in Africa, about one-third of the interviewed women gave these non-numerical responses to fertility preference questions, and others gave unrealistically high ones (Frank 1987). Such responses are problematic for economists using models generating numeric targets for fertility, since it implies that fertility is not a choice variable (Van de Walle 1992). In fact, it implies that people are experiencing a 'natural fertility regime' (Leridon and Menken 1979), defined by an absence of fertility control that depends on parity (although not the absence of *all* control). This means that we should look again at what people think influences their fertility.

Approaching the question from a different direction, it is easy to see that the question 'why children?', or 'how is fertility chosen so as to maximize utility?' only makes sense in a world where fertility falls within the 'conscious calculus of rational choice', and where couples or individuals have a great degree of control over their reproduction, i.e. in a world with available and efficient contraception.[3] The 'Up to God' response should act as a signal to us about the conditions prevailing in the population studied. As Caldwell remarks on its use in Yorubaland (Nigeria):

> This is neither an evasive nor a superstitious reply and such respondents are perfectly happy to discuss what they mean, which is really that these are matters over which they have little control and that to attempt more control would probably achieve little while bordering on the impious. (Caldwell 1982: 21)

The more I thought about these matters, both in Mng'aru and on return to Britain, the more I became convinced of two corollaries. First, that economists, instead of trying to deny the validity of experience behind such responses, should take them seriously by abandoning decision-making explanations of fertility, and concentrate instead on the economic implications of fertility patterns for individuals and households. Secondly, that while it was clear that conscious individual fertility control was largely absent in the area where I was working,[4] fertility was nevertheless controlled, or at least was well below that of other non-contracepting populations. It therefore seemed inevitable that such controls were supra-individual in nature. If this is accepted, then a whole new aspect of the problem is opened up. Once the focus is shifted away from a model where fertility is determined individually through utility or income maximization towards a supra-individual regime of controls on fertility through marriage, divorce, remarriage, breastfeeding practices, taboos on sexual intercourse, polygyny, and other factors, a large number of explanations of fertility behaviour become potentially directly relevant.

The Structure of the Book

Once the approach is accepted, two kinds of study are implied, and both are carried out in this book. One project is the explanation of how fertility (or human reproduction in general) is determined. This is addressed in Part I. Chapters 1 and 2 set out the record of fertility change and the proximate determinants respectively for Rufiji District from about 1920 up to the 1988 census. Chapter 3 examines the main institutional forms involved in the social control of fertility behaviour. Chapter 4 then looks at historical change in Rufiji over the twentieth century, while Chapter 5 offers an analysis of shifts in the demographic regime.

The other project is to take fertility patterns as given data, and look at the resulting structure of families and households and at the consequences for labour roles and patterns. This is done in Part II, and uses questionnaire data

[3] These are the two less considered out of Coale's three necessary conditions for a fertility transition (Coale 1973).

[4] In Rufiji district in 1985–6 about 2.4% of the female population of reproductive age were being supplied with contraceptives, according to figures from the district hospital. My own survey in Ikwiriri implied a contraceptive prevalence rate of between 1.6 and 4.7%.

gathered mainly from one village, at the level of individuals. In Chapter 6 the rural economy of Rufiji in general, and Mng'aru in particular, is described. This is followed by an analysis of accumulation in the village, and its link to household demography, in Chapter 7. Chapter 8 deals with the nature of the life cycle in Mng'aru, and finally Chapter 9 examines the effects of household demography on patterns of work for men and women.

PART I

Introduction to Part I

Over time, the explanation of fertility has been like a mirror image of Karl Popper's model for science. Rather than the discarding of falsified theories and convergence towards a single, elegant explanation, the last thirty years have seen a multiplication of competing approaches. Despite debates which try to settle disputes, proponents of theories rarely give them up—even the demographic transition model, which was looking decidedly ill in the wake of the Princeton European Fertility Project (Coale and Watkins 1986), has recently been revived (Chesnais 1992).

In these circumstances it is perhaps unwise to enter into a theoretical review. However, the approach taken in this book has been the result of a particular view on fertility explanation, and a justification of the approach rests on an explication of that view. Put briefly, the analysis presented here is seen as a contribution to what has been named as the 'political economy' of fertility (Greenhalgh 1990). It is concerned with both global and local histories, and with both structure and agency (ibid. 90). This approach has been taken because it avoids what I see as pitfalls in the many other theoretical formulations. In particular, it avoids the functionalism of 'demand' theories of fertility, and also their lack of attention to the supply or proximate determinant factors. It also avoids the absence of agency in more recent accounts based on cultural structure.

In this introduction I spell out these arguments in detail, and also provide some background to the ecology of the Rufiji area.

Theories of Fertility Change

Early theorizing about reproductive change centred on the question of permanent fertility and mortality decline in a demographic transition (Notestein 1945; Davis 1963). In the post-transitional Western world, fertility levels were seen as the outcome of rational decision-making—the problem was why the rest of the world had not yet moved into the low-fertility phase. Early treatments saw high fertility as an irrational hangover from an earlier type of society where it had originally played a functional role. As modernization proceeded, and mortality fell, it was argued, only cultural and religious 'props' maintained high fertility.

From the 1960s onwards, demographic transition theory came under increasing attack for the two central but insupportable elements which it had inherited from its intellectual genitor—modernization theory. These were firstly the assumption of a move from irrational to rational decision-making, and secondly the notion of a single evolutionary path common to all societies. The result was the development of an array of fertility theories which, although they restated transition theory, ultimately provided only different versions of it.

These versions stressed the rationality of high fertility in pretransitional societies, and most usually in economic terms. What they all have in common is that they explain both high fertility, and the permanent transition to low fertility, in terms of the demand for children. This can be seen in four main schools of fertility theory: neoclassical economics, Caldwell's wealth-flows theory, fertility as insurance against risk, and functionalist Marxism. Since these have been so influential, but are not followed here, some explanation of them, and why they are problematic, is warranted.[1]

Demand theories of the fertility transition

In the initial writings of the 'new home economics', fertility was determined by a demand for children, which was in turn affected by their costs and benefits relative to commodities demanded by a unitary household.[2] Children were in fact treated like other commodities, all of which required inputs of market goods and time, so that the 'price' of children depended partly on the opportunity cost of time involved in rearing them, especially the mother's time. The other part of the model involved an explanation of why, since other goods cannot be substituted for children, fertility nevertheless fell as incomes rose over the twentieth century. This was that parents cared not only about the quantity of children they had, but also about their 'quality'—a reference to the amount of resources, such as education, they would put into rearing each child. Quantity and quality had to be traded off, so that higher-quality children could be obtained only by having fewer children.

Early critics of the neoclassical approach to fertility questioned the choice-theoretic framework. As Griliches put it in an early critique:

> My belief is that if we want to study the demand for children, we have to put more content into the theory, and start asking why do people want to have children; what are the returns and not just the costs of this activity. (Grilliches 1974: 547)

Writers of the school typically just said that children provided 'child services' (Willis 1973) which were both 'monetary and psychic' (DeTray 1976: 185). While unsatisfactory, this at least appeared logically consistent. As De Tray pointed out, economists do not usually worry about the content of utility; 'I suggest that we can contribute . . . significantly to the explanation of household fertility without knowing explicitly why it is that parents have children' (DeTray 1976: 191).

However, even within its own limits, the early new household economics faced problems which led eventually to a shift away from optimal numbers of children as the outcome of decision-making, and stressed instead the roles

[1] The following discussion is a summary of a more comprehensive treatment in Lockwood (1989*a*).

[2] The 'classics' of the new home economics approach to fertility are: R. J. Willis (1973); T. W. Schultz (1974); T. P. Schultz (1976); G. Becker (1981).

that children might play. As Nerlove pointed out as early as 1974, while a family utility function was one of the bases of the approach, it assumed a fixed family composition at the same time as it was supposedly explaining family composition. The only way round this was to incorporate or internalize childrens' interests in their parents' (i.e. the family's) utility functions (Nerlove 1974: 531). This immediately brings in a motivation for the demand for children; the internalization 'which seems so central to the Chicago utility function, has most important implications for the inter-generational transfers of material wealth and human capital' which have been 'so eloquently described as central to the continuity of the social order' (ibid. 532). In fact, this functionalism is to be found implicit even in the original version of new home economics (e.g. Mueller 1976: 145; Becker 1981: Ch. 11).[3]

An important critic of the early neoclassical view which could not see the basis for a demand for children was John Caldwell. In his research in West Africa he could see many reasons. In Caldwell's theory of fertility change, there are only two kinds of stable demographic states. In one, before any demographic transition, economic rationality implies a limitless number of children. Actual fertility, which is high, is determined only by physiological factors. In the other state, after the transition, it is economically rational to have no children at all. Again, actual fertility is determined by non-economic factors—the emotional returns to having children.

The explanation behind this description relies on the concept of 'wealth flows'—all benefits of an economic, political, and social nature passing from one person to another, including goods, money, and most importantly services. In pretransitional societies, the organization of production and exchange along extended family lines—the familial mode of production—means that the net wealth flow between generations is from young to old. By contrast, in post-transitional societies, net wealth flows are from old to young.

[3] The development of intergenerational exchange as an explanation of fertility regimes found its most sophisticated expression in Willis's (1982) attempt to nest John Caldwell's theory of fertility (see above). Essentially, he is concerned with the way in which the older generation seek to recoup some of the costs of raising their children. Central to his model is the idea that children can be invested in, derived from Becker and Lewis's (1974) ideas of 'child quality' and 'human capital', e.g. training and education. The optimal amount of investment will depend on the level of technology in the society, which will also determine the direction of intergenerational income transfer (Willis 1982: 208–9).

There are then two situations which Willis contrasts: a high technology, low fertility society with efficient financial institutions (including pensions), where childrens' economic role is impersonalized; and a low-technology, high-fertility society, where the demand for children is generated in two ways. First, simply, if net transfers of income over the lifetime are from child to parent, the demand can be understood in terms of demand for income (widely defined). Secondly, even if children do not fully pay back the cost of their upbringing, in the absence of other institutions by which resources may be transferred through time, children have value because they fulfil this role (Willis 1982: 225–6).

This is a functionalist explanation in the sense that it is explaining why people have children by one of the attributes or functions of children, and in the absence of any other substantive explanation (Cohen 1978: ch. 9). The shift in economic models of fertility, from children as the object in a unidirectional model of choice to children as actors in an intergenerational model has brought a shift in explanatory emphasis from decision to function.

Transition occurs when two things happen, the implication being that the first is prior. First, the structure of the family economy is transformed from extended to nuclear, and concomitantly the relationships between parent and child are transformed. Secondly, at the wider level, the familial mode of production is absorbed into the capitalist mode of production. Caldwell is very clear that what causes the economic change in the family is *emotional* nucleation, which in turn is brought about through the Westernization of pretransitional societies, via mass education and the mass media (1982: 148–51).

Both high fertility and declining fertility are ultimately explained by virtue of their function in the familial economy. There is an explicit chain of resoning from the maintenance of that economy, and the situational advantage of the male and elderly within it, through demographic decisions (marriage, sexual abstinence) to the beneficial effects of fertility patterns: 'The economic and social structure of the peasant family is focused on the control of familial labour and consumption. Its demography can be fully and satisfactorily explained in these terms' (Caldwell 1982: 163). Thus fertility is determined according to its contribution to given social and economic ends.

One of the elements of benefits from children in pretransitional societies focused on particularly by Mead Cain in the context of South Asia is their role in mitigating risk and providing security for parents in old age (Cain 1981, 1983, 1986). He argues that in the absence of insurance or credit markets, children provide an alternative way of coping with events such as drought, flood, or political crisis, as well as a more permanent source of support in old age. Cain's work has been challenged on theoretical grounds by Nugent (1985), while Vlassoff (1990) has argued that it is not applicable in some South Asian settings. Nevertheless, the idea of high fertility as a response to insecurity remains powerful. Fertility will not fall, on this view, until there are measures to promote social security, or indeed until poverty and inequality are eliminated (Thomas 1991).

The last type of demand-based fertility theory I shall consider is that deriving from classical Marxism. For Marxists, the key variable in determining population processes is the demand for labour, and, since every different mode of production in different periods of history has different laws governing labour demand, 'every special historic mode of production has its own special laws of population, historically valid within its limits alone' (Marx 1970: 592).[4]

Under capitalism, labour demand acts as the conduit for the influence of capital accumulation on population. Like Marx, later theorists such as Coontz distinguished between the early phase of 'primitive' accumulation and the later phase of 'industrial capitalism'. In the former, with a more or less given level of technology (constant organic composition of capital), accumulation is limited only by the number of labourers available. In this period, mercantile capitalism desperately seeks more people:

[4] See also Coontz (1957: 103–4); Gimenez (1977: 7–8, 11, 17).

> [T]he problem of underpopulation is solved by the enclosure movement which 'liberates' the serfs from their instruments of production; and . . . by 'the turning of Africa into a warren for the commercial hunting of black skins.' (Coontz 1957: 111)

By contrast, with the rapid development of industrial technology in the latter phase, labour can progressively be substituted by machinery (rising organic composition of capital). This will tend to happen especially where there is a shortage of labour relative to a particular production process—higher wages induce substitution of workers by machinery, turning a relative underpopulation into a relative surplus population. These workers then form an industrial reserve army of the unemployed (Coontz 1957: 113–17; Gimenez 1977: 7).

This classical story has been augmented by an account of how quantitative and qualitative changes in labour demand may act, at the level of the individual labourer or family, to influence fertility. In a by now familiar way, Coontz traces the economic function of the family in precapitalist modes of production as a 'production and consumption unit' (1957: 190) through to the Industrial Revolution, where the previously domestic contributions of children become material contributions as they enter the industrial labour market. The key to declining fertility at the end of the nineteenth century in Europe is then in the change in the *nature* of labour demanded. This becomes progressively more educated and skilled, taking a longer period of time to 'produce' (ibid. 167, 192–3). The rise in the quality, or average cost, of labour demanded leads to the disappearance of children from the labour force. Other writers, such as Gimenez, in fact see the process as one whereby the way in which household production (and child and female labour) relates to industrial production changes, and changes differently for households of different social classes (Gimenez 1977: 8, 15).

In these accounts of population regimes and fertility changes, fertility is explained by its contribution to the path of capital accumulation, through labour demand (Cootz 1957: 189–93; Gimenez 1977: 16), and ultimately by the dominant mode of production: 'Abstractly considered, reproductive behaviour reproduces the human species. However, if understood concretely and historically, it is a crucial moment of the process of reproduction of all modes of production' (Gimenez 1977: 18).

An application of Marxist demand theory of particular interest here is Cordell *et al.*'s sophisticated approach to African historical demography based on an apparently thorough theoretical understanding of reproduction in Marx and Engels' work. Starting from Engels' definition of what they call 'total social production' as 'the production of both the means of subsistence and of human beings' (Cordell *et al.* 1987: 22), they proceed, influenced by feminist materialist theory, to a separation of three aspects of that production much along the lines described in the Introduction above.

However, as has been noted elsewhere, 'these general statements are not analysed in any depth' (Vock 1988: 93), and when it comes to a lower-level theoretical account of reproduction in Africa under colonial and peripheral capitalism, everything becomes collapsed into a single 'household strategy':

> Production and reproduction occurred within the household or family unit. Production and consumption took place primarily within a larger domestic group . . . The survival and success of the household depended upon its labor: the more people of working ages, the greater the production. (Cordell *et al.* 1987: 24)

In terms clearly echoing post-structuralist anthropology, they go on to specify the function of the 'broader reproductive system' as the maintenance of a 'capacity to renew and recruit productive members' through ensuring 'reciprocity in the exchange of women between lineages' under the control of a 'patriarchal gerontocracy' (pp. 24–5). As Vock succinctly puts it: 'Our understanding of childbearing is reduced to nothing more than the reproduction of labour power' (Vock 1988: 82).

Cordell *et al.*'s account of how capitalist relations of production lead to an increase in the 'pressure for fertility' by the introduction of money and wage labour is strongly reminiscent of Meillassoux's equally reductionist theory, where such circumstances are said to 'favour . . . a burst in natality' (Meillassoux 1983: 50).

Problems with 'demand' theories

The 'demand' approach to fertility explanation has often been criticized, but the critique has made most explicit in the work of John Cleland (Cleland 1985; Cleland and Wilson 1987). Cleland's attack on demand theories is based primarily on arguments from historical and contemporary empirical evidence.[5] The Princeton European Fertility Project provided problems for transition theory more generally, because it showed that fertility decline need not follow that of mortality, and also that fertility decline was not related uniformly to levels of socio-economic development (Knodel and van de Walle 1979). Cleland further points out that historical data provide examples of fertility decline in some areas which are identical in conditions of demand for children to areas where there was no decline (Cleland and Wilson 1987: 16). He uses multicountry World Fertility Survey data to argue that the link between women's economic activity and their fertility is 'obscure' (ibid. 21) and that the effects of female education cannot be reduced to economic effects (ibid. 22). He has further pointed to the relative significance of cultural differences in explaining fertility differentials, between countries (Cleland 1985: 235) and of linguistic or ethnic groups (p. 242). Most recently, he has argued that rapid fertility decline in Bangladesh has little to do with considerations of economic security, but rather is due to an active family-planning campaign combined with an underlying preference for small family size (Cleland 1993).

Cleland's position is disputed, both on grounds of data and interpretation (Robinson 1992; Thomas 1993).[6] One of the problems raised is that Cleland

[5] See also Polgar (1972: 208).

[6] Empirical evidence for the labour and security value of children is also constantly being updated (see Clay and Vander Haar 1993). Indeed, it is undeniable that children contribute more economically at young ages in most African countries than in, say, Britain. But the question is whether that is relevant. Cleland's view is that the economic value of children is largely irrelevant to fertility transition.

has little to put in the place of economic rationality, except inconclusive reference to 'ideational' processes in fertility decline. This reflects a general problem with the eclipse of economic theories and the rise of cultural explanations—what does 'culture' mean? (Hammel 1990).

Nevertheless, Cleland's critique provides sufficient grounds for questioning the empirical validity of economically based demand theories of fertility. It also makes a useful distinction between explaining different *kinds of fertility change*. Much of what he is concerned with is a permanent decline in marital fertility, almost always involving the adoption of modern contraception. But as he points out, this is far from the only kind of fertility change (Cleland 1985: 225). For example, total fertility rates can change because of shifts in age at marriage or marriage incidence (see also Smith 1981). Fertility within marriage can also decline without there being a clear change in stopping behaviour; rather, marital fertility change may reflect shifts in spacing that are not plausibly related to a target number of children. In other words, we need to be able to distinguish between different kinds of fertility determination. Demand theories are precisely problematic because they are implausible except where parents exercise direct and conscious control over marital fertility. This is true only in post-transitional societies, not in pretransitional ones. It is partly for this reason that demand theories are not sufficient for explaining transition itself. As Cleland and Wilson point out, they concentrate on only one of Coale's three conditions for transition—that lower fertility must be advantageous—at the expense of the other two—knowledge and availability of contraception, and that fertility must be within the 'calculus of conscious choice' (Cleland and Wilson 1987: 6).

These distinctions thus demonstrate a second major difficulty for demand theories—their neglect of the 'supply' factors in fertility—in the form of the proximate determinants framework developed in the 1970s and early 1980s (Bongaarts and Potter 1983). This development has shifted interest somewhat away from how socio-economic factors might directly influence fertility towards how they might influence marriage patterns, postpartum infecundability, contraceptive take-up, and so on.

Alternatives to a demand for children?

A central part of the critique brought to bear on demand-based theories concerns the form of explanation and its implications. Firstly, critics rejected the notion of a single transition with uniformly high and homeostatic fertility and mortality on one side, and low fertility and mortality on the other, through which all societies would pass (Polgar 1972: 204; Kreager 1986: 137). Secondly, they especially criticized the notion that an explanation of family size could be based on fixed, numerically specified norms (Polgar 1972: 204; Kreager 1986: 131). Instead of decision (based on function) they stressed structure, which led to the possibility that demographic outcomes or regimes are the result of decisions or strategies followed for ends quite different from economic maximization achieved through demographic means (Polgar 1972: 208; Kreager 1986: 133).

As with Cleland's 'ideational' approach, however, there are problems in trying to formulate a 'cultural' alternative to economically based theories of fertility. One development has been a set of analyses of African demography making extensive use of cultural structures, including the analysis of fertility through lineage and religion (Caldwell and Caldwell 1987), sexuality through kinship structures (Caldwell *et al.* 1989), and birthspacing and reproduction more generally through kinship and systems of production (Lesthaeghe 1989*b*). The problem with these approaches is that they effectively substitute the demands of a cultural system for the micro- or systemic economic demands we saw above.[7] With concepts of social system strongly influenced by British structural-functionalist anthropology, it is not surprising that demographic outcomes are functional to the system. Equally problematic is that social structure is focused on to the detriment of agency. Again, as with the economic theories, cultural functionalism tells us why fertility must change, but not how.

Any approach to fertility explanation which seeks to avoid these problems will need to eschew functionalism, and also provide some account of motivation or agency. Geoffrey McNicoll's work on institutional approaches to fertility (1978, 1980) has tried to provide general accounts of motivation, although as he himself points out, attempts to theorize institutions often have a tendency to 'persuasive *post hoc* reasoning' (1980: 449).[8]

An example may make the problems faced appear clearer. At first sight, an excellent model for the kind of fertility explanation suggested by the discussion here would be Randall and Winter's (1985) analysis of fertility differentials in Mali between two groups of nomadic Tamasheq and agriculturalist Bambara. The former groups have much lower fertility than the latter, but this can almost entirely be explained by differences in marriage patterns. Tamasheq women marry late and reluctantly, and divorce readily, so that they spend a great deal of their time out of sexual union. This is turn explained convincingly by the instability of marriage in a strongly matrilineal kinship system, where women identify more with their brothers' interests than with their husbands'. Husbands are willing to divorce women because they do not need their labour in a pastoral production system. By contrast, Bambara women marry early and have a low divorce rate, live in a patrilineal system, and are central to food production and agriculture. Husbands seek to secure a wife early and hang on her because of her labour value (Randall and Winter 1985: 159–60).

The weakness is in the latter, Bambara, part of the story. The argument may be correct in this case, but it is not convincingly so. This may be seen in a comparison with Hausa demography. In Nigeria Hausa women marry when they are young, and remarriage is high. Like the Bambara they are settled agriculturalists at the upper reaches of the West African savannah. However,

[7] For a detailed discussion see Lockwood (1995).

[8] See also Bardhan (1989).

unlike Bambara women, Hausa married women are largely secluded and are not involved in agricultural fieldwork. There is no *necessary* connection between early marriage and female economic value. Randall and Winter's study is exemplary in its comparative method, its tracing of fertility differentials through the proximate determinants, and its reference to local institutions. However, at the end it falls back into an argument based on economic rationality.

By comparison, the two benefits offered by an anthropological political economy are, first, a balance between structure and agency, and, secondly, recognizing the importance of history (Greenhalgh 1990). These are benefits because both are powerful corrosives of abstract asserted models. However, the requirements for obtaining these benefits are considerable, involving both detailed historical research and anthropological fieldwork. The analysis presented in this book falls considerably short of such ideals, partly because of the difficulty of reconstructing history in a place such as Rufiji. Nevertheless, if a journey is to end in a particular destination, it helps if the first steps are taken in the right direction.

Consonant with this approach, Part I attempts a preliminary political economy of fertility change in Rufiji. Chapter 1 assesses the evidence for change in fertility. There is evidence for little movement in the decades before 1950, but a steady rise thereafter. Nevertheless, fertility in Rufiji and the Coast Region remains below that in other areas of Tanzania. The fertility regime was and is characterized by high levels of sterility, marital instability, and long birth intervals. In Chapter 2, information on the proximate determinants of more recent change is examined. Declines in sterility have played a major part, but so have increases in age at marriage, and possibly a decreasing birth interval. An interpretation of the social and political institutions in which these proximate determinants are embedded is sketched in Chapter 3. It is argued that marriage patterns were closely related to political and spatial organization, while gender relations within marriage are crucial to an understanding of marital instability and shifts in post-partum abstinence and breastfeeding. Major elements of change in Rufiji over the twentieth century are described in Chapter 4, while Chapter 5 attempts to provide a synthesis of demographic change with social and economic transformation. At each of these stages, arguments are highly circumspect, limited by the scanty and defective nature of historical data which need careful and constant interrogation.

Much of Rufiji's history has been dominated by its ecology. As a final preliminary it is therefore essential to have a broad picture of the regimes of rainfall, flooding, and soils in the district.

An Introduction to Rufiji

Rufiji is an anomaly. Part of the great sweep of the East African coast, or *Mrima*, it shares many characteristics of the numerous other coastal societies which stretch from northern Kenya to southern Tanzania. It is heavily Muslim, and cultivation centres on rice, coconuts, and cashews. It is also, like many other coastal areas, relatively poor and undeveloped, compared with some Christian up-country regions of Tanzania and Kenya. And yet Rufiji is also different, not least because the Rufiji River has cut the area off by land from other parts of the coast, as well as providing a local pole of cultivation and transport. The river floods every year, sometimes covering the floodplain to a width of seven miles.

The river gives the District its geographical, agronomic, and social shape, dividing it into the central floodplain, terraces and hills to north and south, and flowing into the delta on the Indian Ocean coast in the east. The floodplain, 5–10 km. wide for most of its length, extends over 80,000 hectares, and is bounded to the north and south by terraces, leading to hills reaching a height of 300 m. In the south these are the Kichi and Matumbi Hills, in the

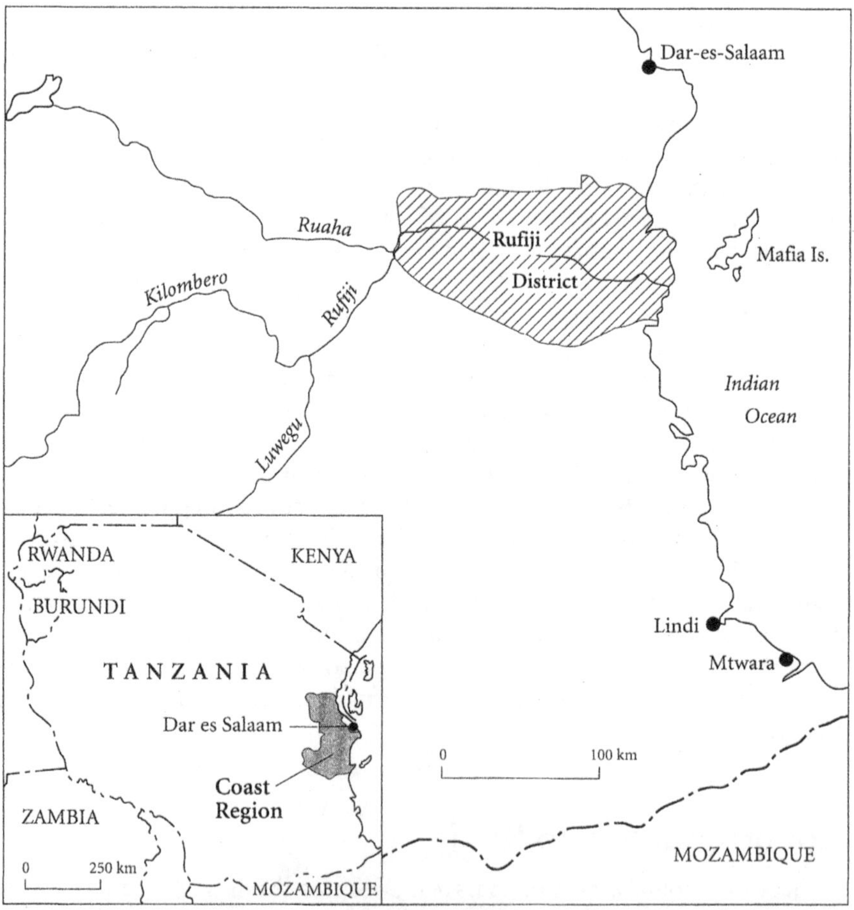

Map 1 *Location of Rufiji District*

north, the Magongo Hills. To the east, the river fans out into a delta on the Indian Ocean coast. There is a bitumen road from Dar es Salaam as far as Kibiti at the edge of the Magongo Hills, about 150 km. south of the capital, completed in 1968.

The broadly defined zones of the flood valley, hills, and delta form distinct ecological systems (Havnevik 1983: 13). The delta to the east of Mohoro is tidal, and as a result of salination and silting only a rather narrow range of activities are possible within it: coconut palm cultivation, mangrove pole cutting, and fishing. The delta has a aura of dread for many Europeans: in the First World War the German warship *Koenigsberg* was hit and damaged off the coast and forced to go to ground in the channels of the delta. Attempts were made to repair it there, but it was spotted by the first air flight made in Tanzania, and soon after destroyed. The wreckage is still visible. To Commander Villiers, writing during the First World War campaign in Tanzania, this was a terrible environment: 'If in this world there is a worse place than the Rufiji delta, I hope to God I may never find it. The whole delta is gloomy, morose and depressing beyond belief.'

Nevertheless, the delta was for a long period the richest area within the district, since it was until the 1930s the nexus of all trade with Dar es Salaam, and the heritage of this wealth is still apparent today. More than other parts of the district, the delta remains a world largely apart from the rest of the mainland.

The hill and floodplain systems, with which this study is more concerned, are both primarily agricultural, but quite distinct. In the hills and terraces, sandy, mildly acidic, and moderately fertile soils predominate, with poorly drained clays in depressions (Cook 1974: 8–9; Havnevik 1983: 24). The hills experience slightly less rainfall than the lower floodplain, and are good for drought-resistant crops: cassava, pigeon peas, sorghum, millet, and cashews. In the depressions, which normally become water-logged during the long rains (see below), rice, maize, and cotton have all been grown. In addition, a wide variety of fruit and vegetables can be grown, including coconuts, citrus fruits, and pulses. The geomorphology of the floodplain is by comparison more complex, since it is partially reformed every year to a greater or lesser extent by sedimentation from the floods. The resulting great diversity in soil type and quality brings an element of variation to agriculture in the floodplain. This is, moreover, compounded by the interaction of rainfall and flooding regimes.

Bantje argues that rainfall and flooding are the two dominant environmental factors in the floodplain: in good years complementing each other to bring about excellent conditions, especially for rice; in bad years bringing either drought or damaging floods, or even both (Bantje 1979: 20). In the hill ecological system, much the same can be said of rainfall alone.

Mean annual rainfall figures show that rainfall declines with westward movement through the district. Even where there is moderate rainfall, however, such as Utete, on average four out of ten years show insufficient rainfall and in the west there is even more variation, frequently leading to drought and crop failure (Bantje 1979: 22; Havnevik 1983: 17–18).

Monthly rainfall figures show that there are effectively two rainy seasons (Cook 1974: table 3.1; Havnevik 1983: table 2). In fact, the agricultural year can be divided into three phases on the basis of rainfall patterns (Bantje 1979: 20). The short rains, usually occurring during October and November, correspond to the *vuli* growing season of October to January. The timing of these short rains is crucial, since it determines the start of agricultural activity, with the preparation of fields (Bantje 1979: 22), while their quantity and duration determine the success or failure of early food crops. This then sets the conditions for the second period, from February to May/June, which includes the long rains, and the floods in the valley. This season produces the main rice and second maize crop. The third season, from June to October, is essentially a dry season, but in the valley a further crop (often cotton or maize and pulses) can be obtained after heavy flooding. This is known as the *mlao* or *mlau* crop, whereby the roots of the crops planted in innundated areas follows the falling water-level (Telford 1929; Bantje 1979: 1; Havnevik 1983: 22).

Because of the temporal and spatial variability of rainfall, flooding is important for crop water requirements in the valley. In addition, floods are beneficial in that they increase soil fertility and maintain the delta ecological system (Yoshida 1974; Bantje 1979: 24–5; Havnevik 1983: 18). At the same time, excessive floods can do immense damage to crops, property, and life. The flood regime of the Rufiji is created by rainfall and run-off in the catchment area of the river and its tributaries. This determines the timing, duration, and quantity of the floods, which in turn produce the specific effects of the flood on agriculture and communications (Bantje 1979: 24). Early, high floods tend to wash away rice seedlings, while late, low floods do not provide enough water. Equally, short, well-timed floods, even if very high (e.g. as in 1969) can produce excellent crop results, while slightly lower, but long-lasting floods (e.g. six months in 1968) can be very damaging.

There are also differences in flood effects by location. Floods arise quickest and highest in the upstream portion of the floodplain; by the time Mohoro is reached, the flatter valley and run-off to lakes makes the flood more gentle and so less destructive. Finally, variation in field elevation in the valley, between depressions and levees, means that crops on lower fields can be washed away, while those on higher fields give excellent results; or alternatively that in low-flood years lower fields give good yields while higher fields face water shortages.

The interaction of topography, soil variation, rainfall, and flooding in the valley gives rise to what Bantje (1979: 26) has called 'excessive variation' in agricultural production, essentially requiring a detailed micro-ecological knowledge of seed varieties, planting times, flood resistance, and water requirements to ensure a good yield.

The great uncertainty in agriculture in both valley and hills, and the complex production systems devised to minimize this uncertainty, have had considerable consequences for political and domestic organization in the district. These factors are of central importance in understanding the demographic history of the district.

1 The Historical Demography of Coastal Tanzania

By the standards of historical demography where long series of registers or other records exist, either in Africa or elsewhere,[1] writing a demographic history of Rufiji means becoming a detective faced with a minimum of clues. There is an inverse relationship between the specificity of the reconstruction and its distance in time from the present.

Approaches to the demographic history of Tanzania have changed considerably over the last forty years, as have ideas about demographic change in Africa as a whole.[2] In the early post-Second World War period, demographic transition theory was important, based on the assumption that all countries would follow Western Europe through a series of demographic changes in the course of 'modernization'. Pre-industrial birth and death rates were held to be high, but fell as economic development progressed. Mortality was thought to have fallen first, followed by fertility, giving a burst of growth in the early period of transition. However, the historical basis of transition theory was shown to be unsound by the Princeton European Fertility Project: countries with different levels of economic development experienced transition at the same time; fertility in pre-industrial settings was neither uniform over time, nor always high (Coale and Watkins 1986).

In Africa, it was assumed that pre-colonial fertility and mortality were high, giving the low growth rates which explained the relatively sparse population of a large continent. Colonization was believed to be followed by a population boom as fertility lagged behind falls in mortality made possible by the 'benefits' of colonial health services. However, with the questioning of demographic transition theory, and the expansion of both demographic and historical sources, a number of new ideas were introduced into the demographic history of Africa. In the East African context, a key work was Helge Kjekshus's (1977) revision of the history of the precolonial and early colonial period. Contrary to the conventional view that Tanzania was beset by high mortality through famine and war in the late pre-colonial period and then benefited from 'Pax Brittanica', Kjekshus argued that pre-colonial Tanzania was a relatively stable

[1] For examples of the availability and uses of records from Africa see Fetter (1991) and *African Historical Demography*, vols. 1 and 2, Centre of African Studies, University of Edinburgh. See also Cordell and Gregory (1980). For a contrasting example of the records used in English historical demography see Wrigley and Schofield (1981).

[2] See Fetter (1990: 5–9) for a more comprehensive account.

and safe environment which was ravaged by disease, war, and social disruption in the course of conquest and pacification. Mortality rose sharply and did not fall considerably until well into the century, on this view.[3]

The other new idea was that fertility in Africa, and in Tanzania, had actually risen over the colonial period. The rise of fertility during the colonial period concurred with evidence from India, where sources were better, and was taken up as a central point by Marxist demographic historians of Africa (Meillassoux 1983; Cordell *et al.* 1987). In Tanzania, the importance of rising fertility has been argued for by Turshen (1984) and Koponen (1986). In this Chapter I examine each of these issues in turn, focusing on Rufiji as far as the existing data allow.

Precolonial and Early Colonial Population Change

Of the issues debated in East African demographic history, there is one on which all commentators agree. This is that there was a drastic decline in, or at least a stagnation of, population from the mid- to late-nineteenth century up to the 1920s (Culwick and Culwick 1939: 30–2; Kuczynski 1949: 395–6; Kjekshus 1977: ch. 1; Hartwig 1979: 654; Iliffe 1979: 123). At a national and East African level, it is also agreed that this was ultimately accelerated by an ecological catastrophe from the 1890s onwards, involving rinderpest, locust plagues, trypanosomiasis and sleeping sickness, sandfleas, famine, influenza epidemics, and two major wars (Culwick and Culwick 1938: 375; Kjekshus 1977: 69, 126, 132, 134–42; Iliffe 1979: 123–5, 159, 161, 165, 199–200, 269; Patterson 1981: 408–9, 421).

The major controversies in this demographic history concern the growth of population and levels of mortality in the pre-colonial period, from the 1840s and 1850s to the 1890s. The extension back in time of arguments concerning high *colonial* mortality has been most recently made by Juhani Koponen. He argues that: 'Mortality in the late pre-colonial and early colonial period seems to have been exceptionally high, and it is difficult to estimate what the more 'structural' pre-colonial mortality levels might have been' (Koponen 1986: 39).

The point has been made more polemically by Hartwig, in a direct riposte to Kjekshus's (1977) extended thesis of 'minimum population disruption' in precolonial Tanzania. Kjekshus argues that the localized famines and skirmishes reported by early travellers do not constitute evidence for a serious population crisis through famine and war in precolonial East Africa, especially when compared with the collapse that was to follow 1890. Hartwig disputes this, invoking Kuczynski, who compiled a demographic survey of the British colonial empire at the end of the Second World War, to his support (Hartwig 1979: 654–6). At other points, however, Kuczynski appeared to pour

[3] The view that population in East Africa declined in the late nineteenth and early twentieth century was first put forward by Kuczynski (1949: 119).

scorn on the argument that mortality was excessively high in East Africa before colonial conquest (Kuczynski 1949: 118–20).

Part of his assessment involves an interesting argument about the sociology of European perception of African population trends. Colonial observers overestimated nineteenth-century mortality due to famine and internecine warfare, and they tended to believe that population had declined from a previously higher level because the total population in the mid-nineteenth century was not that large—they assumed that East Africa had become depopulated (Kuczynski 1949: 118, 120). This tendency to judge the East African situation purely in comparison with the contemporaneous western European demographic experience also encompassed fertility. Early nineteenth-century travellers, used to the high fertility rates of Britain, stressed the relatively low fertility of African societies. However, by the late nineteenth century, colonial officers who were accustomed to falling marital fertility in western Europe began to emphasize the high-fertility societies they came across in East Africa.

At a general level, these arguments about precolonial levels of mortality and population are impossible to resolve without further data. As Hartwig puts it:

> A satisfactory assessment of demographic patterns in East Africa during the nineteenth century is premature. Our assembled knowledge is still too meager to identify the important variables, let alone determine the impact they might have had. There are also very important regional differences. (Hartwig 1979: 656–7)

This suggests that more-localized studies are of greater value, and the remainder of this chapter therefore concerns the sequence of demographic events in the locality of Rufiji and the coastal areas of Tanzania.

The standard account of precolonial Rufiji is one of almost legendary abundance. This is based on the argument that the delta and floodplain had a large population supported by the successful export of food surpluses and other goods to the nearby coastal centres:

> We should remember that the city formation of the East African coast dates back several centuries, and that string of townships in varying stages of prosperity included Bagamoyo with 25,000 inhabitants in 1889, which besides Kilwa Kivinje with 15,000, Tanga, Pangani, Sandani, Lindi and Zanzibar, must have added up to a considerable demand for foodstuffs. This demand caused reverberations in a number of agricultural areas near the coast and stimulated their specialisation as grain and vegetable suppliers for the urban centres. It seems likely that part of the flat and enormously fertile river valleys in the south were particularly affected by these developments. (Kjekshus 1977: 30)

> In 1811 [Zanzibar] was already drawing rice from the Mrima. Sixty years later the Kisiju area specialised in growing manioc to feed slaves awaiting shipment from Kilwa. Mwera grew millet and manioc for export, and the Rufiji valley—which Stanley declared the most populous area he had ever seen in Africa—was so famed for its rice that the delta was known as Little Calcutta. (Iliffe 1979: 71)

> The export of large quantities of foodstuffs (beans, maize, rice and sesame seeds) from the Rufiji villages to Zanzibar was recorded by Zeigenhorn. His review indicated

> relatively heavy population concentrations near the fertile flood plains where the main villages were located. Indigenous food demands must have been considerable. The agricultural production in most villages aimed, however, beyond self-sufficiency to create a considerable surplus for export outside tribal boundaries. (Kjekshus 1977: 31)

Kjekshus also cites Marsland's 1938 assessment of the Rufiji as a 'veritable agricultural Eldorado', and Elton's 1874 account of a journey from Mohoro to the Rufiji river as a three-hour march through a 'land of plenty'.

Bantje, however, has argued that this favourable picture must be qualified in two ways. Firstly, he emphasizes the important ecological and agricultural differences between the upstream area and the downstream and delta area—the former experiencing much greater variation, and hence more risk of flood and famine. This partly explains the 'Rufiji paradox: while the famous large harvests are mainly produced downstream, the famines mostly occur upstream. Even in very good crop years food shortages have sometimes occurred in the upstream villages' (Bantje 1979: 26).

Secondly, in his historical review of famines and floods in the district, he has found records of early famines going back before the 1890s. As early as 1877–80, combinations of drought and heavy flooding caused minor famines in the downstream areas. This was repeated in 1884 (Bantje 1980: 3–6).

However, as at the national and regional level, local events took a severe turn for the worse only after 1890. The arrival of rinderpest in 1891 had little effect in Rufiji, since it was not a major cattle-keeping centre. Smallpox, however, was epidemic in this period, killing off an estimated one-tenth of the population of Dar es Salaam in 1893 (Iliffe 1979: 124). The first component of the ecological catastrophe of the 1890s to have a major impact in Rufiji was an infestation of locusts in the mid-1890s, leading to protracted famine. The 1890s were also extremely dry, and the failure of rains in three successive seasons led to a further famine in 1898–1900 (Bantje 1979: 1–2; 1980: 3–6).

These events were only a prelude. As Iliffe notes, the ultimate agent of ecological crisis in southern Tanzania, involving the spread of tsetse fly, massive famine, and disease, was the MajiMaji War (Iliffe 1979: 164). German troops deployed a crop-burning strategy to break the rebellion, forcing surrender through famine, and bringing about an estimated 200,000–300,000 deaths. The Rufiji area was particularly affected (ibid. 165, 199).

Fewer than seven years passed before another wave of ecological and demographic disaster passed over the area. A series of epidemics afflicted the district during the First World War, beginning with bubonic plague in 1914; then cerebro-spinal meningitis in 1916; influenza in 1918–19; and smallpox in May 1920 (TNA 1733/1; RH, 1937; Kuczynski 1949: 326; Patterson 1981: 408–9).

In addition to the direct effects of the war, in which only 3,000 of over 15,000 men drafted as porters returned to the district, there was a major famine in 1917. Localized famine triggered by drought occurred in Rufiji again in 1924–5 and in 1929–30, the latter causing substantial emigration from the district (RH, 'Notes on Census'; Bantje 1980: 3–6).

Thus, up until well into the 1920s, it was clear that a number of serious environmental, political, and epidemiological crises had militated against the growth of the population, or even caused a decrease. Contemporary and slightly later sources seem to concur in identifying a fall in population. Colonial officers in the 1920s and 1930s took the view that population in Tanania generally had been falling since before 1885 up to 1920 (Kuczynski 1949: 395–6). In Rufiji, the decline was attributed to epidemics, endemic malaria, hookworm and yaws, emigration, famine, slave-raiding, and high infant mortality (TNA 1733/18: 105; RH, 1937).

Part of the evidence of depopulation was that large numbers of mango groves could be seen scattered through the forest in the west of the district—these were taken to be signs of long-deserted villages (RH 1937). It is not clear if this can be taken at face value. Cross-Upcott's work on the Wangindo implied that much of Rufiji society was spatially mobile, so that deserted villages or hamlets need not denote depopulation (Cross-Upcott 1956). This is disputed, however, by Kjekshus who contrasts Cross-Upcott's account of a mobile forest-based people—only recently so according to Kjekshus—with Decken's nineteenth-century description of Ungindo as heavily and permanently settled (Kjekshus 1977: 73–4).

Equally unclear is the demographic significance of some of the ecological catastrophe components. For example, historical work has brought a reassessment of the demographic significance of famine, suggesting its effects may be less severe and more age-selective than is conventionally supposed (Watkins and Menken 1985). Part of my argument in Chapter 5 below is that demographic slowdown may have also been partially due to a disruption of marriage patterns brought about by the political crises of wars and famines.

However, all the evidence before the 1920s points to serious dislocation of economy and society, and to population stagnation and decline in the previous thirty-five years. The elements of this situation were low fertility and high mortality, and were particularly in evidence in Rufiji and the other coastal areas.

Relatively low fertility in the area can be observed in its legacy of a low child/adult ratio for the 'Warufiji' in the 1931 Census. Compared with the relatively more fertile groups at this time, such as Wachagga and Wanyakusa, the Warufiji child/adult ratio is near the bottom of the national scale (Kuczynski 1949: 351). More directly, there are reports of low fertility specifically in the coastal areas from medical and other colonial officers (TNA1733/1, Dar es Salaam and Kisarawe; Kuczynski 1949: 378–9). This has been further confirmed by more recently appraised evidence from the German period (Koponen 1986: 42). By comparison, mortality was relatively high and probably changed little even up to the 1940s (Culwick and Culwick 1939: 30–2; Kuczynski 1949: 119).

Kuczynski argued that the demographic turning point for Tanzania occurred in the mid- to late-1920s. While in the early 1920s people were still suffering the after-effects of the war, the second half of the 1920s saw some improvement (Kuczynski 1949: 319, 398). In particular, as instability decreased, the latter half of the 1920s saw an improvement in medical services for the general population. In Rufiji an apparently successful campaign against yaws and widespread vaccination against smallpox were instigated in

1925 (TNA 1733/18: 105). In addition, famines, although still frequent, had less disastrous consequences as countermeasures became more organized. Progress was stalled in the 1930s as expenditure on health services was curtailed by the financial effects of the Depression, and it was not until after the Second World War that investment in services resumed (Kuczynski 1949: 382; Koponen 1986: 40). Despite plans as early as 1924 for a district hospital, services and investment in the 1930s in Rufiji were completely lacking (TNA 61/3/VI/D).

Population Growth in Colonial Rufiji

Quantitative estimates of the population of Rufiji become available early in the twentieth century. However, as with other British and French colonies in Africa, no proper censuses were taken until just before or after Independence in the late 1950s and 1960s.[4] Earlier estimates were of two kinds. First there were assessments based on the number of taxable adult men. In colonial Africa it was a common practice to raise this figure by a multiplier to derive an estimate of the total population. Numbers of children and women were derived according to certain fixed proportions. In early years of administration, these proportions were set at what were thought to be reasonable levels, and in later years were often based on a small 'sample' of a few villages in a territory or region. In Rufiji, the proportions of adult men to total population over the period from 1921 up to 1948 lie between 0.15 and 0.19. The exception is 1928, when the proportion is 0.23. These multiplying-up factors were probably too small. By 1957, with the most complete census so far conducted in Tanganyika, and despite substantially greater post-war male out-migration to Dar es Salaam, the ratio of adult men to total population in Rufiji was 0.2008.

A second basis for estimation was a count of total population. This is distinguished from a census in that record is made of total numbers of people rather than enumeration of details of individuals. In neighbouring countries, such as Zambia, which like Tanganyika had tiny numbers of administrators and enumerators relative to the population, such counts were done by gathering male heads of households together, and asking them about their families. In the absence of particular men, village chiefs were asked (Stone 1990).

These figures are thus characterized by a range of inaccuracies and biases, and are typically undercounts. They are especially unreliable with regard to the non-taxed part of the population, i.e. women and children. Combined with the fact that the distinction between adults and children was unreliable and often arbitrary, this state of affairs led the colonial demographer Kuczynski to the conclusion in 1948 that 'knowledge of the age composition therefore is practically nil' (Kuczynski 1949: 102). However, some information is better

[4] See the collection of papers on Belgian, French, and British colonial territories in Central Africa in Fetter (1990), especially that by Stengers.

than none at all. The total population figures from these counts, district estimates, and later censuses for Rufiji District are shown in Table 1.1. These figures are adjusted for boundary changes, as described in Appendix 1.1. For some years there are two estimates, these figures having been compiled from various sources.

The unreliability of these figures is evident in their erratic nature. Year-to-year variations of up to 4,000 people in a population of around 70,000 (i.e. over 5 per cent) are highly implausible. This is so even if traumatic events, such as famine, are taken into account. For instance, while there was famine in 1929–30 (see above), recorded at the time as causing movement of people out the district, which might explain the sharp drop in the total for 1931 from the District Books, the 1931 Census gives a figure almost 8,000 higher, for the same year.

Table 1.1. *The population of Rufiji District, 1913–1988*

Year	Population	Year	Population
1913	*78,337*	1931*a*	69,961
1921	*83,200*	*1931b*	*77,864*
1925*a*	76,852	1948*a*	101,349
1925*b*	78,601	*1948b*	*107,296*
1927	70,256	1951	116,340
1928a	*74,037*	*1957*	*118,458*
1928*b*	74,686	*1967*	*121,024*
1929*a*	73,845	*1978*	*135,334*
1929*b*	74,394	*1988*	*152,316*

Note: Figures in italic are official census or count figures.

Sources: See Table A1.1.

Table 1.2. *The population of Rufiji District, 1913–1988* (selected estimates)

Year	Total population	Growth rate (% p.a.)
1913	77,337	—
1921	83,200	0.75
1928	74,037	−1.67
1931	77,864	1.68
1948	107,296	1.89
1957	118,458	1.10
1967	121,024	0.21
1978	135,342	1.02
1988	152,316	1.18

Source: See Table A1.1.

To obtain a more stable indication of growth rates, only the more widely spaced official census and count figures have been used in Table 1.2, i.e. those in italic in Table 1.1.

The first point to note is that these estimates are not net of migration, which probably grew up to 1945, and certainly after that date (see below). Thus the underlying growth of the population from the late 1920s to 1957 is probably understated. On the other hand, later counts, and the censuses from 1948 onwards, are probably progressively more complete, so that recorded growth may not reflect real growth. Given this, the overall impression is that population growth in Rufiji was relatively low throughout the period, and apparently very low or non-existent before the Second World War.

Mortality and Fertility in the Mid-Twentieth Century

Demographic data for Tanzania become more reliable and plentiful with the advent of modern census-taking in 1957. However, much of the interesting data, especially on fertility, is useful at the regional rather than at the district level. Rufiji District lay in Eastern Province, and later in the Coast Region. Provincial and regional data are thus partly a reflection of the district picture, but are also formed by the broader context of demographic processes in eastern and coastal Tanzania.

Migration

Since the establishment of settled communities in Rufiji there has probably been a trickle of migrants, going and returning to and from the city states of the coast. Certainly from the late nineteenth century onwards, migration to other parts of Tanzania and East Africa was well established. It was not until after the Second World War that Dar es Salaam dominated as a destination. Although it was chosen to be the capital and main port of German East Africa as early as 1891, the city grew only slowly up to 1945.

Equally important destinations for early migrants were Mafia and Zanzibar, and for those in the southern part of the district, Kilwa and Lindi (TNA 61/3/VI/D; RH, 'Report on Censuses'). Zanzibar played an especially important role, not only as an economic pole of attraction, but also as a cultural and religious one. The Rufiji District Book reports in 1937 that 'Zanzibar is [a] favourite place for emigrants, and it is reported that there are six villages there holding more than 3,000 people from this district.'

After the inter-war years of the slow growth of the African labour force in Dar es Salaam, the Second World War and the years that followed saw an unprecedented increase in urbanization. According to census figures, the total population of the city increased from 69,277 in 1948 to 272,515 in 1967 (Sutton 1970: 19), reflecting an average annual growth rate of over 12 per cent.

Early migration from Rufiji (and elsewhere) to Dar es Salaam was predominantly male. This can be seen not only in high sex ratios for Dar es Salaam (Bienefeld and Sabot 1972: Table 3.9), but also in the decline of the Rufiji adult sex ratio in the early post-war period (Table 1.3). While it has reached a floor in the more distant valley and upstream areas, it seems to be rising again in the more populous and accessible northern area.

In the early post-war period, coastal migrants predominated in the growth of the city. The initial relative importance of coastal migration for the growth of Dar es Salaam has lessened over time. Table 1.4 shows the place of birth of residents of Dar es Salaam at different times. As can be seen, in the immediate post-war period, up to one-third of those living in the city had been born in the surrounding area. As late as 1967, the proportion was still about one-quarter. In that year, 35 per cent of migrants to Dar es Salaam came from Coast Region, and in 1971 the National Urban Mobility, Employment and Incomes Survey of Tanzania gives the figure as 24 per cent (Bienefeld and Sabot 1972, vol II: Table 4.1; 1967 Census; Egerö 1974: 42). However, by the late 1970s the proportion had fallen, squeezed not only by flows of migrants from elsewhere, but also by the growing proportion of the population (i.e. children) who had been born in Dar es Salaam.

Mortality

Mortality information for Tanzania prior to the post-independence national Censuses is patchy and of varying quality. Various sources give the infant mortality rates (IMRs) shown in Table 1.5. There has been considerable debate

Table 1.3. *Sex ratios, Rufiji District, 1921–1988* (no. of males per 100 females)

Year	Total	<16	>16
1921	93.3	104.9	87.1
1927	91.3	97.2	88.8
1929	96.5	96.9	96.2
1931*a*	97.7	115.5	90.3
1931*b*	101.0	116.5	94.5
Early 1940s	97.5	—	—
Second World War	98.5	—	—
1948	82.1	104.6	69.9
1949	89.2	—	—
1957	87.1	93.9	82.6
1967[a]	84–8 (V)	—	—
	92–4 (N)	—	—
	84 (U)	—	—
1978	89.8	—	—
1988	94.4	—	—

[a] V = valley area; N = northern area; U = upstream area.

Sources: 1921–31, 1948, 1957—Lockwood 1989*b*: table A1.6; 1940s, Second World War, 1949, 1967—Bantje (1980: 13); 1978, 1988—census volumes.

Table 1.4. *Place of birth of Dar es Salaam residents 1952–1977* (%)

Place of birth	1952	1956[a]	1967	1977
Dar es Salaam	25.9	30.3	30.6	36.0
Coast Region	—	—	23.8	17.0
Kisarawe District	18.7	23.5	—	—
Rufiji District	10.0	9.5	(13.5)[b]	—
Other	45.4	36.7	45.6	47.0

[a] Refers to African population of Dar es Salaam alone.

[b] Total percentage of African private households headed by members of the Rufiji peoples (Rufiji, Ndengereko, Matumbi).

Sources: 1952, 1956—Leslie (1963: table 3); 1967, 1973, 1978—censuses.

over mortality decline in colonial Tanganyika. Turshen (1984: 46–47) argues that mortality by the 1940s and 1950s was still high—higher than Blacker's (1963) estimate of a CDR of 24–5 per 1,000 in 1957. She offers an alternative figure of 35 per 1,000. This argument implies that mortality did not fall substantially in the prior period, Turshen quoting Kuczynski's view that fertility must have been higher than commonly was supposed. Kuczynski (1949: 119) did argue that mortality had not in fact decreased much between 1900 and 1940, but on the other hand he also saw contemporary estimates of mortality as far too high. With an infant mortality rate of 500 per thousand, he points out (p. 124), even very high fertility rates could not have brought about the assumed 1.5 per cent p.a. rate of natural increase for Tanganyika. He argues that growth in the 1940s was probably lower (about 0.5 per cent) and a 'reasoned guess' at the infant mortality rate was not exceeding 250 per thousand. The figures in table 1.5 suggest that up to the 1940s only slight improvement in mortality had been made, and it was only by around 1950 that the IMR begins to fall below 200 per 1,000. However, it should be noted that estimates for 1957 and onwards were different in nature from earlier ones, being derived from techniques introduced by Brass at this time.

But more systematic estimation of national trends in fact supports the picture given above. Unpublished work by John Blacker and William Brass (Brass n.d.) obtains retrospective estimates of the probability of death by exact age 5 (q(5)) from the five censuses between 1948 and 1988, plus the 1991–2 Demographic and Health Survey. These estimates indicate that the under-5 mortality rate was over 300 per thousand until 1950, after which it began to fall quite sharply to about 170–90 per thousand by 1980.

A more systematic picture of trends for the Coast Region and for Rufiji District can also be obtained, using methods of mortality estimation originally devised by William Brass. Information on children ever born and children surviving from recent censuses can be used to produce estimates of mortality

Table 1.5. *Infant mortality rates, 1913–1991/2* (per 1,000 live births)

Year	Infant mortality rate
1913	230
1921	300
1927	284
1928	271
1929	263
1941	243
1947	254
1948	170
1957	193
1967	145–160
1967 (Coast Region)	127
1978	135
1988	115
1991/2	107

Sources: 1913, 1948, 1967, 1978—Koponen (1986: table 2.1); 1921, 1927, 1928, 1941—Kuczynski (1949: 392 (Kilimanjaro), 394 (Kahama), 395 (Ngeza); 1947—Martin (1953); 1957—Coale (1968); 1967 (Coastal Region)—Sembajwe (1984); 1988—Census Infant and Child Mortality: Regional and District Estimates; 1991/2—Tanzania Demographic and Health Survey (Coastal Zone).

projected back in time (UN 1983: ch. 3).[5] Applying this technique of mortality estimation to data from the 1967 Census, the 1973 *National Demographic Survey* (*NDS*), the 1978 Census, and the 1988 Census, trends in child mortality for Coast Region can be produced, dating from about 1950 up to the mid-1980s (Fig. 1.1).

In interpreting these series, it is important to bear in mind that they are produced by a technique which has quite restrictive assumptions. In particular, they are based on an assumption of steady change in mortality, so that the estimates are not sensitive measures of short-term fluctuations, but rather should be looked at for longer-term trends (UN 1992: 7). In addition, the estimates for the youngest age group (15–19) are considered unreliable and biased, and are not included in the graph.

Taking the period from 1950 onwards first, mortality trends in Coast Region appear somewhat different from the national picure. Levels of q(5) in the early 1950s, according to the 1967 Census data, are in the range 0.22–0.24, compared with a national range of 0.26–0.29. Thus while child mortality in the mid-1980s ends up at around the same level as the national average (0.18–0.2), the

[5] See also Brass (1975: ch. VIII; 1985: 2–10, 17–32). Here, the estimates of q(5) use the 'North' variant of the Coale–Demeny model life tables.

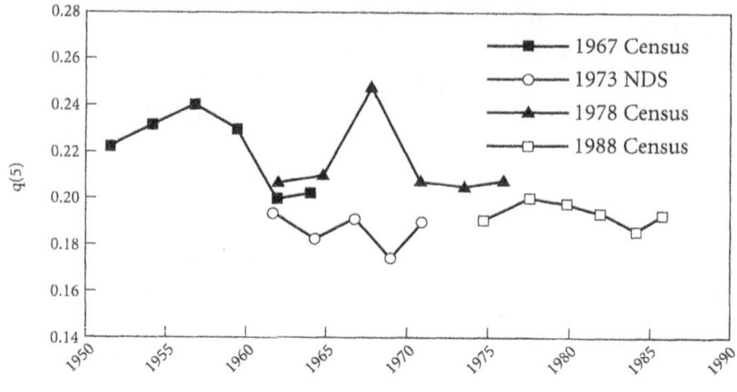

Fig. 1.1 *Child mortality: Coast Region*

apparent fall off is much less steep. The data from the three censuses in 1967, 1978, and 1988 are broadly consistent, with the exception of the high figure in the middle of the 1978 series. The 1973 *NDS* data appear to underestimate mortality.

The 1991–2 Tanzanian Demographic and Health Survey also provides us with some recent estimates of mortality. The TDHS was a sample survey, and the smallest area for which published figures are available is the 'coastal zone', which covers four eastern mainland regions plus Zanzibar. The survey gives a figure of 107 per thousand for the infant mortality rate in the period 1981–91, close to the 1988 census estimate. But the direct estimate of q(5) is much lower, at 0.1603. This difference (also observable at national level) could be due to differences in the questions asked between census and survey.

Overall, these figures imply that there had been only slow progress in reducing mortality in Coast Region between 1950 and the 1980s, relative to national movements. However, there are reasons for doubting this conclusion. Data from the 1957 and 1948 Censuses suggest much higher levels of infant and child mortality around the beginning of this period. Brass and Blacker have used national data on infant deaths and average parity for broad age groups from these early Censuses to model survivorship and mortality rates (Brass n.d.). The 1948 census gives an 'infant wastage rate'—the proportion of children dying under age one from all live births—of 0.1717 for mothers aged 13–45. This generates a q(5) estimate of about 0.31 in the mid-1940s. Similarly, a wastage rate of 0.192 for 16–45-year-olds in the 1957 census gives a q(5) estimate of around 0.33, located in the early 1950s. For the Coast Region, the 1948 and 1957 infant wastage rates for the 16–45 age group are 0.183 and 0.222 respectively, while the average parities are similar to the national figures.

All of this suggests that the 1948 and 1957 census data point to much higher levels of q(5) for the Coast Region in the 1940s and early 1950s than is indicated by the 1967 series (i.e. in the range 0.3–0.35). The regional data are in any case less stable than the national data, with less agreement between series, but an underestimation of child mortality in the older age groups for the 1967

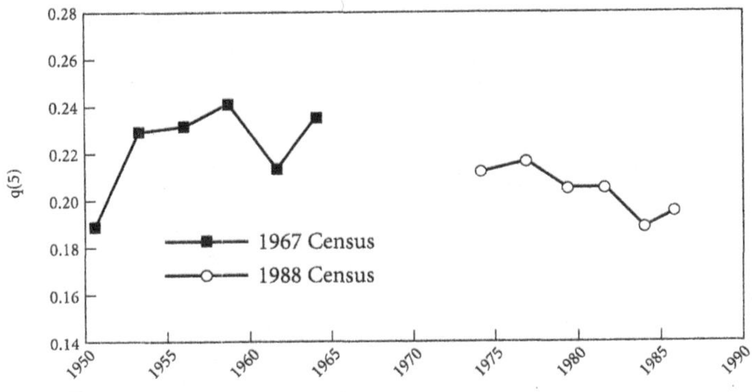

Fig. 1.2 *Child mortality: Rufiji District*

Census also seems likely. However, it can certainly be said that both the Coastal and the national figures, even at the higher range given in the earlier censuses, support Kuczynski's argument that the child death rate was nearer 0.3 than 0.5 in the 1940s. Data for mortality estimates at the district level are available only from the 1967 and 1988 Censuses (Fig. 1.2). The trends roughly mirror the regional data, but the estimates are more erratic, especially for the earlier period.

Fertility

Perceptions of a slow fall in mortality in late colonial and post-colonial Tanzania led to arguments that fertility must have risen significantly over the century to produce accelerating population totals (Turshen 1984: 48; e.g. Koponen 1986). It in fact appears that the rise was particularly steep in other areas of Tanzania, notably in the highlands and the West Lake area (Koponen 1986; Brass 1987). The rise in Rufiji, and in the Coast Region generally, was more modest in the sense that when comparable census fertility figures become available, coastal fertility is relatively low—the lowest in the country outside of Dar es Salaam region. Period fertility rates from published Census sources imply rising fertility in the post-Second World War years (Table 1.6).

However, a more detailed picture of fertility change in the coastal area can be obtained from a technique which again projects information in recent Censuses back in time. An application of this technique is available in Feeney (1988), on which the analysis here is based. The basic idea is to look at the completed fertility patterns of older cohorts. A first step is to look at data on mean children ever born (MCEB). Following Feeney (1988: 7. 1.20), women of 40–4 and upwards are considered. Since this cohort has not quite completed fertility, the most recent figure for each series will be slightly lower than the true MCEB. However, the difference is likely to be very small. Again, despite the assumptions built into the technique, it is useful for the investigation of trends.

Trends in children ever born for the Coast Region (and for Eastern Province in the 1948 and 1957 Censuses) are shown in Table 1.7. The data are of

Table 1.6. *Period total fertility rates, 1948–1991/2* (births per woman)

Year	TFR (recorded)	TFR (adjusted)
Mainland		
1948	—	5.0–5.1
1957	—	5.6–6.4
1967	7.3	6.6
1973	—	6.3
1978	6.4	6.9
1988	—	6.5
1991/2	6.59	
Coast Region		
1967	5.8	4.9
1973	—	5.1
1978	6.1	5.3
1988	5.47	—
1991/2[a]	5.7	

[a] 'Coastal area' includes Coast, Morogoro, Tanga, Dar es Salaam Regions, plus Zanzibar.

Sources: 1967, 1978, 1988—censuses; Koponen (1986: 33); 1973—*National Demographic Survey*; 1991/2—DHS.

Table 1.7. *Mean children ever born, Coast Region/Eastern Province*

Birth cohort of women	Year of census or survey					
	1948	1957	1967	1973	1978	1988
Before 1908	4.1	4.76	4.15			
1909–13		3.58	4.01	3.87	4.8	
1914–18		4.99	3.82			4.04
1919–23			3.91	3.61	4.5	4.35
1924–8			3.70	4.15	4.7	4.35
1929–33				4.05	4.6	4.87
1934–8					5.2	5.29
1939–43						5.81
1944–8						5.79

Sources: 1948, 1957, 1967, 1978, 1988—Census volumes. 1973—*National Demographic Survey*.

uneven quality, those for 1957 being particularly erratic. There is some evidence of improving completeness of reporting, especially between the 1967 census and 1973 *NDS*, and the 1978 and 1988 Censuses.

Secondly, and perhaps most importantly, while there is clear evidence in the table for rising fertility for cohorts born after the mid-1920s (corresponding to rising fertility from about 1950 onwards), there is no evidence for such a trend before that date. Indeed, there is a trend of slightly falling fertility, most clearly in the 1967 Census. The pattern for the whole country is not dissimilar, with mean completed births remaining roughly constant up to about 1950, albeit at the higher level of around 5.75, before rising to 7 by the 1970s (Brass n.d.). This pattern was noted much earlier in the 1957 census, where comparison of MCEB between the 1948 and 1957 Censuses led to the conclusion that 'it can . . . reasonably be assumed that the general level of fertility had remained fairly constant for some years prior to the 1957 Census' (Tanganyika 1957: 87).

These results may be contrasted to Feeney (1988: Fig. 1) which shows a strong pattern of rising fertility in Kenya from 1915 to 1955. It is noteworthy that for the 1978 data, the MCEB for the youngest age group (40–4) is higher than that of the next age group (45–9). This is unusual, since the former group have not quite completed their fertility. It is thus a sign of rising cohort fertility.

For a more detailed understanding of what has been occurring we must turn to parity progression ratios for the Coast Region over the period. Parity progression ratios (PPRs) are defined as the ratio between the number of women in a group (here a cohort) having at least $(n + 1)$ children and those having at least n children. Thus, for example, the PPR from 1 to 2 is the ratio of those with two or more children to those with one or more, and so on. PPRs have been used as particularly sensitive indicators of changes in fertility behaviour, especially parity-specific fertility behaviour (Feeney 1988).

The PPRs for Coast Region for the period from the 1930s up to 1960 are shown in Fig. 1.3a–h. The dates of PPRs are derived from assuming that child-bearing of a cohort was concentrated in one year, when the women were 25 years old. This is clearly an artificial device, but can be understood as locating a date as being at the centre of the fertility distribution over the lifetime (Feeney 1988: 7.1.20). The PPRs are derived from the 1973 *National Demographic Survey* and the 1978 and 1988 Censuses. Unfortunately, published data for constructing PPRs from the 1967 and earlier censuses are not available at the regional level. For most of the PPRs, the 1978 and 1988 sources agree better than the 1973 *NDS*, which tends to understate parities. It is also clear that the different sources are consistent for the lower order PPRs, and then start to become erratic and less smooth at the higher-order parities.

However, given the limitations of these data, we can consider some points about the ways in which fertility trends for Coast Region have evolved. A preliminary point is that the PPR graphs generally support the notion that there has been little parity-specific fertility control in the Coast Region. With the exception of the erratic movements in the higher-order PPRs in the 1973 data, there are none of the sharp drops characteristic of the adoption of early stopping behaviour.[6] Most of the PPRs up to quite high parities lie close together, although they start relatively low. The PPRs from 1 to 2 for Kenya were

[6] The exceptions discussed could be due to small numbers, and also to the fact that it is the highest parities where the incompleteness of the 40–45-year age group's fertility is most apparent.

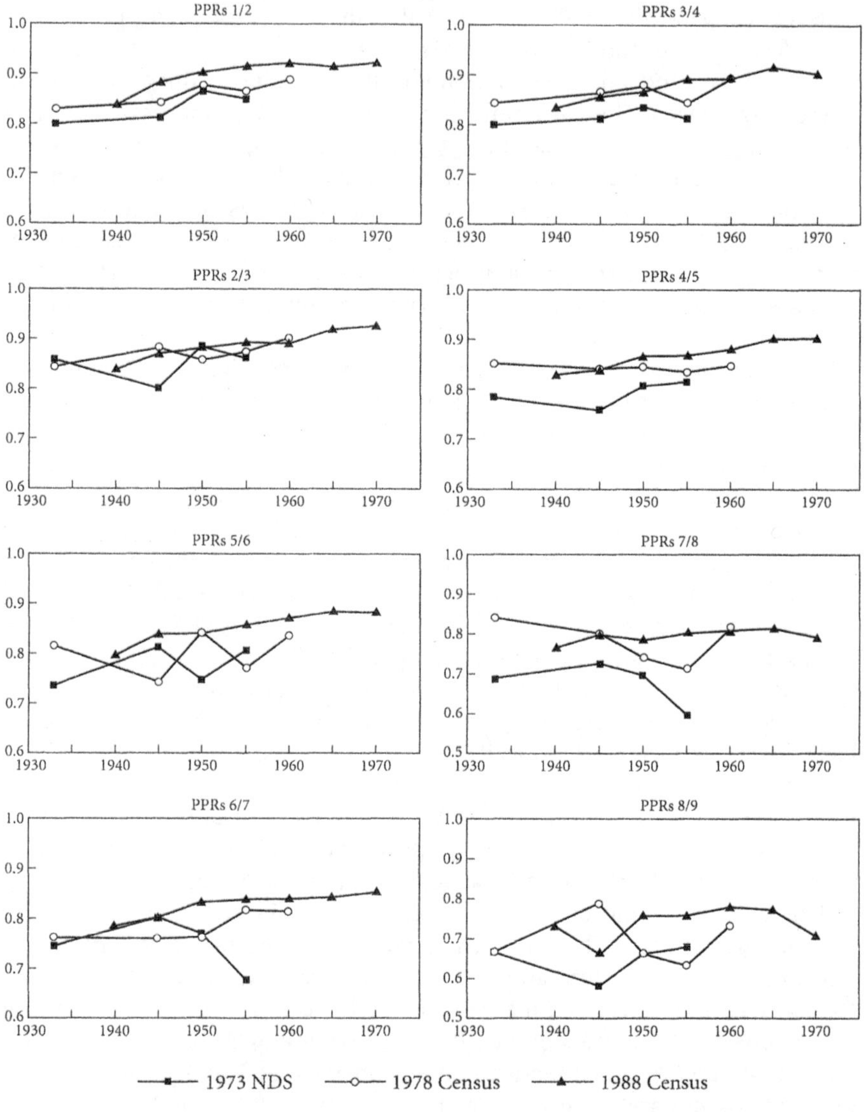

Fig. 1.3 *Parity progression rations: Coast Region*

between 0.93 and 0.96; for the Coast Region these ranged from 0.8 up to about 0.92. This suggests higher levels of secondary sterility in the latter area (see Chapter 2 for further discussion of sterility).

How did this change over time? Up to parities of 6 or 7 the PPRs show a drift upwards across the whole period, but especially after 1950. Higher parties show little change. As in Feeney's Kenyan data, this may suggest a change which is tending to contract most birth intervals by a similar amount. These trends are consistent with the rise in MCEB after 1950 observed in Table 1.7, but is somewhat at odds with the lack of increase in MCEB earlier than that. However, given the robustness of the PPR measures (e.g. Brass 1985: 71), it is likely that this pattern of sustained change from an earlier date is closer to the truth.

The relatively low level of the 0 to 1 and 1 to 2 PPRs in comparison with the Kenya data, together with the marked increase in parity progression ratios for lower parities, raises the issue of infertility trends. Table 1.8 shows the proportion of women aged 40 and over with no births (indicating primary sterility) and one or two births (indicating secondary sterility).

While these data strongly suggest a decline in primary and secondary sterility over the century, there are clearly problems with the consistency of the series. This is especially so with the very high figures for older cohorts in the 1988 data, a pattern also seen in the national data, and attributed by Brass to difficulties with the 'not stated' category (Brass n.d.).

All the data above imply that fertility has been rising in the Coastal area of Tanzania, as in the rest of the country. The rising trend in parities is clearest in the most recent data set, the 1988 Census. The data from these reconstructions take us up to 1970. Adjusted total fertility rate estimates from the 1967 Census, the 1973 NDS, and the 1978 Census imply that the upward trend in fertility continued through to the late 1970s and possibly beyond. Only in the 1988 Census and the 1991–2 TDHS are there indications that the trend in fertility might have peaked.

One further way to approach more recent fertility trends is to extend the parity progression ratio analysis further in time, using Brass's P-F synthesis (Brass 1985: 69–73).

PPRs for younger cohorts will be biased because of truncated fertility histories. Thus, while younger women will already have had some children, which gives us their distribution by parity, we do not know their future fertility behaviour. However, what we can do is to show what would happen if they were to follow the fertility behaviour of their elders, given by their parity-specific cumulated fertility, $F(i,j)$, for the ith age group and the jth birth order. Adding parity and fertility elements together gives us predicted fertility by birth order, from which it is possible to derive a set of PPRs, which are synthetic in the sense that they represent a combination of actual and predicted fertility behaviour.

The only 1988 Census Coast Region data available for calculating the parity-specific current fertility element of these synthetic PPRs were in the form of the proportion of women with births in the last year, which did not specify the *number* of births to those women. For the vast majority of women, those giving birth in the last year will have had only one child. However, a few may have had a very short birth interval, or more likely multiple births (twins, triplets, etc.). The extent to which the current fertility of each age group is thus underestimated can be checked by comparing the sum of the proportions of women with births in the last year across birth orders with the number of children born to women in the age group. This shows an underestimation of fertility in the order of 5 per cent, except for the youngest and oldest age groups, which are in any case of less interest. In fact, since we are looking at changes

Table 1.8. *Percentage of women with 0 and 1–2 births, Coast Region/Eastern Province*

Birth cohort of women	Year of census or survey									
	1948		1957	1967	1973		1978		1988	
	0	1–2	0	0	0	1–2	0	1–2	0	1–2
Before 1908	14.4	22.0	13.1							
1909–13			26.5		16.6	22.1	10.7	17.1		
1914–18			16.8						25.8	19.0
1919–23				16.9	16.9	29.2	10.5	24.1	22.0	18.7
1924–8					14.9	20.2	11.7	22.0	24.2	18.3
1929–33					13.2	23.3	9.2	21.9	19.1	16.8
1934–8							9.0	18.0	16.7	16.5
1939–43									12.0	14.1
1944–8									11.0	13.0

Note: Data for 1978 are rural.

Sources: 1948, 1957, 1967, 1978, 1988—Census volumes. 1973—*National Demographic Survey*.

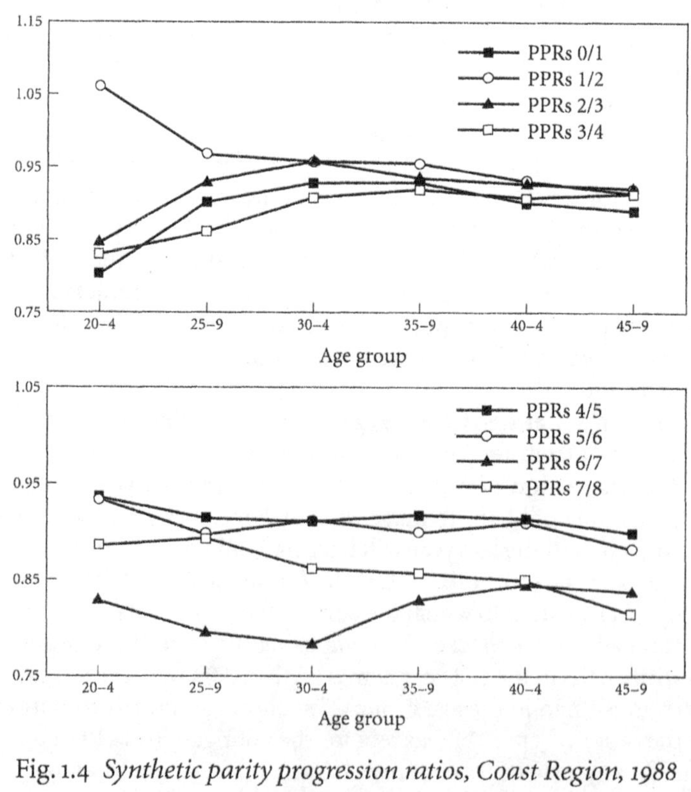

Fig. 1.4 *Synthetic parity progression ratios, Coast Region, 1988*

across time rather than absolute levels of fertility, the fact that the underestimation is similar across the age groups of interest means that the comparison based on these data is broadly valid.

These PPRs are shown in Fig. 1.4. The projected element is largest for the youngest age groups, and thus is the least accurate for these age groups. The technique is most useful for comparing the oldest age groups, for which the synthetic PPRs are nearly the same as achieved PPRs, with the middle age groups. If there were a sharp decline in fertility in the Coast Region in the late 1980s, we would expect to see movement in the PPRs of this middle group. As can be seen in Fig. 1.4, there is no evidence for such a change. The PPRs for lower parities are quite smooth (with the exception of PPR 1 to 2 for 20–24-year-olds) and show, if anything, a slight increase for middle as compared with older age groups. The higher-order PPRs lie less close together, but only that for 6 to 7 shows signs of falling off in the middle-range age groups. In any case, these higher-order PPRs are less stable, as they are based on smaller numbers of births than the lower-order ones.

Conclusions

This examination of the principal qualitative and quantitative sources on the demographic history of Rufiji District and its coastal environs has led to a number of findings.

Firstly, there was almost certainly a stagnation or decline in population during a period of social and ecological crisis between 1890 and 1920, although the absence of any quantitative data means that this remains speculative. The elements of this were high mortality and possibly lower fertility.

Secondly, child mortality in the Coast Region and in Rufiji probably fell from a q(5) in the region of 0.3–0.35 in the 1940s to around 0.2 by 1970, and to below 0.2 by the late 1980s. Kuczynski's case for an infant mortality rate of 250 per thousand for the 1940s is plausible, if a little on the low side.

Thirdly, fertility in the Coast Region was stagnant or possibly rose slowly throughout the period 1930–1950, and has almost certainly risen since 1950. The rise in fertility has continued up through the 1980s. However, overall levels of fertility on the coast are low relative to the rest of Tanzania.

The analysis of data on demographic change in coastal Tanzania provides the starting point for the first half of this book. Focusing in on the changing patterns in fertility, the next four chapters explore the setting and causes of those patterns. The next step in that exploration is to look at the proximate, or biosocial determinants of fertility.

Appendix 1.1. The Population of Rufiji District 1913–1988

The available figures are shown in Table A1.1.

These raw figures, however, require a number of adjustments because of administrative boundary changes and the reassesment of counts. In particular, by 1928 the 1913 German count was judged to be an overstatement, and the figure for all of Tanganyika was reduced from 4,145,000 to 4,063,000 (Kuczynski 1949: 327). Adjusted figures for districts were not given, so the most we can do is make a proportional reduction in the 1913 figure for Rufiji:

$$\left(4.063/4.145\right)\cdot 89{,}100 = 87{,}337.$$

As Kuczynski notes (1949: 326), the 1913 and 1921 counts are not immediately comparable, because the earlier count includes Mafia Island while the latter one does not. In fact, examination of the administrative history of Mafia shows that up to 1916 it was included in Rufiji, from 1916 to 1919 it fell within Zanzibar, from 1926 to 1930 it was a subdivision of Dar es Salaam, from 1930 to 1951 a subdivision of Rufiji again, before becoming a separate district in 1951. Thus in the census/count years 1913, 1931, and 1948, Mafia was included in the Rufiji total, while in 1921, 1928, 1957, and after it was not. These shifts thus make some adjustments necessary. Kuczynski (ibid. 326) obtains an estimate of Mafia's population in 1913 as 9,500. However, the population of Mafia in 1951 is given as 8,473 (TNA 61/504/1/II). A slightly declining or stagnant population on Mafia would be likely if there were heavy out-migration to Zanzibar and Dar es Salaam over this period. In the absence of any other information, I subtracted 9,000 from those figures for the years in which Mafia was included within Rufiji's administrative boundaries. This yields the adjusted figures shown in table A1.2.

Table A1.1. *Unadjusted estimates of the population of Rufiji District, 1913–1988*

1913	*89,100*	1931a	79,461
1921	*83,200*	*1931b*	*87,364*
1925*a*	76,853	1948*a*	110,349
1825*b*	78,601	*1948b*	*116,296*
1927	70,256	1951	116,340
1928a	*74,037*	*1957*	*118,458*
1928*b*	74,686	*1967*	*121,024*
1929*a*	73,845	*1978*	*135,334*
1929*b*	74,394	*1988*	*153,938*

Note: Figures in italic are official Census or count figures.

Sources: 1913, 1921—Kuczynski (1949: 327); 1925, 1927, 1928*b*, 1929, 1931*a*—District Books; 1928*a*, 1931*b*—Tanganyika, *Census of the African Population 1931* (n.d.); 1948—Tanganyika, East African Statistical Department, *African Population of Tanganyika Territory* (1950); 1951—TNA 61/504/1/II; 1957—Tanganyika, East African Statistical Department, *African Population Census 1957* (1958); 1967—Egerö and Henin (1973); 1978—United Republic of Tanzania, Bureau of Statistics, *Population Census, Preliminary Report*; 1988—Preliminary Census Volume.

Table A1.2. *Adjusted estimates of the population of Rufiji District, 1913–1988*

1913	*78,337*	1931a	70,461
1921	*83,200*	*1931b*	*78,364*
1925*a*	76,852	1948*a*	101,349
1925*b*	78,601	*1948b*	*107,296*
1927	70,256	1951	116,340
1928a	*74,037*	*1957*	*118,458*
1928*b*	74,686	*1967*	*121,024*
1929*a*	73,845	*1978*	*135,334*
1929*b*	74,394	1986	146,849

Note: Figures in italic are official Census or count figures.

Sources: See Table A1.1.

2 The Proximate Determinants of Fertility

In Chapter 1 we saw that the available evidence for Rufiji, and the Coast Region of which it is a part, pointed to stagnation of fertility up to around 1950, and a rise thereafter. In the attempt to understand this pattern, the first step must be to identify the immediate or proximate biosocial component causes producing it.

Many economic and sociological studies of fertility seek to relate socio-economic variables (such as income, education, religion, etc.) directly with fertility rates. However, these variables can only affect fertility through certain biological and behavioural factors. The first attempt to codify these relationships came with Davis and Blake's classical 1957 study. On the basis of a thorough modelling of the reproductive process, and greater empirical knowledge of the dimensions of the variables, a comprehensive framework has now been developed of the proximate determinants of fertility, i.e. the biological and behavioural factors which stand directly 'next to' fertility:

> The principal characteristic of a proximate determinant is its direct influence on fertility. If a proximate determinant changes, then fertility necessarily changes also (assuming the other proximate determinants remain constant), though this is not necessarily the case for a socio-economic determinant. (Bongaarts and Potter 1983: 1).

The proximate-determinants approach is based on identifying factors which bear on the various stages of the reproductive process: exposure to sexual intercourse; the probability that coitus will lead to a conception; and the probability that a pregnancy will result in a live birth (Lesthaeghe *et al.* 1981: 4; Bongaarts and Potter 1983: 4–5).

Proximate determinants can be grouped together in various ways, according to the interests of the analysis or types of population. Here I will first distinguish the 'exposure' set of determinants from the others. Of the latter type, the most important are the prevalence of contraception use and abortion, fecundability (monthly probability of conception), the incidence of primary and secondary sterility, and the risk of spontaneous abortion. During the period we are interested in, and even up to the present, Tanzania was an almost completely non-contracepting society. It had, in fact, a natural fertility regime, so that parity-dependent fertility control was absent, although some abortion of socially undesirable pregnancies may have been practised. The important non-exposure determinants are therefore the incidence of sterility and intrauterine mortality, and the frequency of intercourse.

Of the 'exposure' determinants, there are those limiting the overall period of exposure (i.e. usually to within some form of marriage union), and those affecting exposure within marriage. Lesthaeghe has argued that, for sub-Saharan Africa, it is useful to group proximate determinants in this way when seeking to analyse the economic and cultural roots of fertility change. Thus he juxtaposes

> changes with respect to (1) union formation and dissolution, or, in other terms, with respect to the overall exposure time (starting and stopping, loss of exposure owing to union disruption); and (2) the pattern of child spacing mainly operating via lactational amenorrhoea and post-partum abstinence. This duality is essential for several reasons. First, . . . sub-Saharan organisational systems generally favour a maximum exposure span, but correct this via the child-spacing obligation: the two sets of variables act in opposite directions on fertility. Second, the variables delimiting *overall exposure* and those producing *child spacing may have highly different elasticities with respect to cultural or economic influences*. In other words, differential degrees of resistance or erosion of the overall exposure variables and of the child spacing ones results in synthesizing new 'uneven' forms of demographic transition. (Lesthaeghe 1986: 218)

Following this advice, we can group together on the one hand evidence on divorce and female age at first marriage, and on the other hand post-partum abstinence and breastfeeding. Given the evidence on fertility patterns in Chapter 1, there are two main issues. The first is to identify the relative importance of the different factors in determining fertility in Rufiji and the coast, and, in particular, why it has been relatively low. The second is to specify what was responsible for the upward trend in fertility in the post-war period.

The Record up to Independence

Before 1967 there is virtually no quantitative evidence on these proximate determinants.[1] Only the barest outlines of the main factors can be drawn. However, what evidence there is supports Lesthaeghe's division of proximate determinants in Africa. Taking overall length of exposure first, early female marriage was the norm, and although divorce was common, and may have increased between 1920 and 1950, remarriage, or the formation of new sexual unions, was also frequent. Exposure within unions was strongly influenced by spacing factors, notably post-partum sexual abstinence and long lactation. While there is some ethnographic evidence that the former declined over the period, there is none that the latter did. To these standard 'exposure' determinants must be added two others, both of which may have played an important role in depressing the level of natural fertility in Rufiji. One was a high level of stillbirths due to malaria or work stress. The other was sterility due to venereal disease, which may have peaked in the early to mid-colonial period, and declined after 1950.

[1] Except possibly divorce, through primary court records. Owning to time constraints, I did not attempt to examine these.

The 'nuptiality valve' of early modern Europe, with late marriage and high proportions never married, was completely absent in coastal Tanzania (and much of Africa (Lesthaeghe 1980)). Marriage in Rufiji, as well as in nearby areas such as Kisarawe, Ungindo, and Pangani, was universal and early (TNA 1733/1 (Dar es Salam and Kisarawe); Cross-Upcott 1956: 198; Roberts and Tanner 1959: 75; Swantz 1986: 33). Marriage in Rufiji, as in these other areas, was a process often spread over several years rather than an event, and the real point of interest here is the start of exposure to conception. Thus, while child marriages were common, and pre-menarcheal intercourse possibly occurred, the return of the bride to her parents' home and seclusion at menarche leading up to the final rituals of marriage formed an age 'buffer' delaying the onset of exposure (RH, 'Marriage'; Cross-Upcott 1956: 198–209; Swantz 1986: 33).

The duration of seclusion has declined over time, from a number of years to often a nominal one or two weeks, but within this trend, the period also depended upon the transfer of money and goods from the groom's to the bride's family and upon political stability, so therefore upon the absence of famine and war, and the opportunities for wage labour (Cross-Upcott 1956: 208–9). Offsetting the decline of seclusion, there is some evidence of a later average age at first marriage for women, although this only becomes better-documented after the Second World War (Roberts and Tanner 1959: 75).

While union formation was early and universal, observers of Rufiji and other parts of the coast frequently remarked on the instability of marriage by the 1920s and after (TNA 1733/1 (Dar es Salam and Kisarawe); TNA 1733/17/1/10; TNA 1733/18: 105; Roberts and Tanner (1959: 66)). One of the main shifts underlying what was seen as an increase in divorce was the progressive replacement of pre-existing family law by Islamic *sharia*, which was used by both men and women in response to their changing expectations of marriage (TNA 1733/17/1/10; Roberts and Tanner 1959: 75–6; Tanner 1962: 70–1). Another cause was the tax placed by the colonial authorities on polygyny, which led to increased divorce rates in crop-failure years (TNA 1733/5; TNA 1733/18: 105).

A third factor determining overall fertility—the incidence of sterility—attracted by far the most attention in contemporary accounts. By the 1960s and 1970s, Central and East Africa had been identified as major areas suffering from pathological sub-fecundity, mainly due to tubal occlusion caused by gonorrhoea and pelvic inflammatory diseases (Belsey 1976: 326–9; Frank 1983: 138). This was accompanied by secondary sterility caused by post-partum and post-abortal infection or injury.

It is argued that endemic pathological sterility became established after a initial wave of epidemic venereal disease, linked to contact with outsiders through trade, slaving, and wars, up to and including the First World War (e.g. Turshen 1984: 137; Pearce 1986: 86). By the late 1930s, for instance, the Culwicks' study of fertility in Ulanga district showed a generation of older women, whose childbearing years coincided with the MajiMaji and First World Wars, with a high incidence of primary and secondary sterility—35 per cent of these women had less than two children (Culwick and Culwick 1938/9: 373–4).

Once established, infertility was frequently linked by colonial and other sources to promiscuity, and this was thought especially common on the coast. This was, however, disputed by the Medical Officer of Dar es Salaam, who attributed low fertility to abortion and male sterility due to hydroceles (TNA 1733/1; Kuczynski 1949: 378); Roberts and Tanner 1959: 79; Allen 1981: 18).

The relative prevalence of venereal disease after 1914 and the consequences for sterility are difficult to elucidate. Despite alarm about a great increase in venereal disease after First World War, there was in fact no evidence of this (Kuczynski 1949: 326, 378). In 1923, a report on venereal disease favourably compared most of rural Tanzania with Uganda (TNA 19153/I/4). What did undoubtedly increase, starting with the German administration, was colonial concern about venereal disease, as well as about medical policy in general (Beck 1977: 28; Vaughan 1991: 129–54). Venereal disease and related infections were fairly amenable to direct treatment, and by 1929 over 100,000 people had been treated for syphilis as an adjunct to the anti-yaws campaign, including in Rufiji (TNA 1733/18: 105; Titmuss 1964: 5; Beck 1977: 33). Health education continued through the 1930s, culminating in a number of measures during the Second World War which reflected the alarm of the administration over endemic venereal disease (TNA 19153/I/19, 35, 52; TNA 19153/II/5, 12, 14, 36A).

Nevertheless, it is important not to overestimate the effects of medical policy. Much effort was apparently directed towards eradicating syphilis, which in its chronic form is not a major cause of infertility. Campaigns against gonorrhoea did not get under way until way after the Second World War. As late as 1948, the incidence of childlessness in Tanzania was around 17 per cent, and the coastal region had a rate above the national average (Pearce 1986: 3–5, 13). A study in Pangani in the late 1950s showed that the proportion of infertile marriages was still high (Roberts and Tanner 1959: 69). Thus, while the incidence of sterility may have declined from an early colonial peak, it remained an important limit on fertility (see Chapter 1 above).

The other non-exposure determinant of relevance is the probability of bearing a pregnancy to full term. The few individual reproductive histories from this period that include stillbirths point to their appalling frequency (Swantz 1986: 33). However, although the patterns of work stress in rice cultivation probably intensified over the early twentieth century, nothing further can be said about intrauterine mortality with any confidence.

The last two factors affecting fertility through post-partum non-susceptibility—sexual abstinence and lactational amenorrhoe—are probably of prime importance, while at the same time being very little understood or documented. What evidence there is confirms the national, regional, and continental assessment of a decline in abstinence, leaving breastfeeding practices as the major determinant of birth intervals (Schoenmaeckers *et al.* 1981; Bongaarts *et al.* 1984: 522; Koponen 1986: 43; Lesthaeghe 1986: 227).

Early descriptions of coastal post-partum abstinence link it to breastfeeding, and this practice survived into the 1950s for the people of Ungindo (Cross-Upcott 1956: 121–2; Allen 1981: 10). Elsewhere however, abstinence was eroded to an Islamic-influenced forty-day period (Roberts and Tanner 1959: 79). In Rufiji, the representative of UMATI (the Tanzanian family planning body), observed that the arrangements of separate sleeping areas for lactating women and their husbands no longer applied.[2]

By contrast, a long period of breastfeeding and associated post-partum amenorrhoea is still the norm in Tanzania. It is possible that its duration has, if anything, increased. Early reports of partial weaning of infants at three months or less on to *uji* (porridge) in Rufiji and elsewhere prompted attempts at health education for later weaning in the 1930s (TNA 1733/18: 105; Culwick and Culwick 1939: 34). Currently, partial weaning in Rufiji starts at about six months.

The net effects on birth-spacing are observable from a comparative study of a coastal area and one in Kilimanjaro. For the cohort of women who started childbearing from about 1940, those on the coast had a long birth interval of around four years. The comparable figure for Kilimanjaro is 2.79 years. Later cohorts of coast women have experienced shorter birth intervals, but still longer than their contemporaries in Kilimanjaro (Ngallaba 1972: 136). The 1991–1 DHS gives a median birth interval of 34.6 months (2.88 years) compared with 33.3 months for Tanzania as a whole.

It is impossible to attribute relative quantitative or indeed qualitative importance to these determinants in producing a low level of natural fertility. Contemporary observers highlighted the role of venereal disease, but the overall picture was probably more complex.

On the one hand, post-partum abstinence behaviour may have changed over this period, and female age at first coitus (completion of marriage) may have fallen in the 1920s. These factors would have worked to increase fertility. On the other hand, marital instability—i.e. divorce—increased, and venereal disease and sterility remained high. It is not automatically clear that the first factor would depress fertility, since divorce in Rufiji and the coast is not synonymous with the end of exposure (Roberts and Tanner 1959: 78). However, it probably did often mean a period of greatly decreased frequency of intercourse initially. Also, since women often sought divorce on grounds of desertion for a substantial period, the divorce event could equally be a belated sign of decreased exposure.

The Proximate Determinants since the 1960s

From the 1960s, enough census and survey data become available to attempt a rough quantitative assessment of the proximate determinants. This is based on the approach developed by Bongaarts and Potter (1983). They divide the seven determinants into two groups—principal and secondary—according to their importance in most populations. They find that marriage, post-partum infecundability, contraception, and abortion account for most varia-

[2] Interview with Mzee Kilingamoyo, Ikwiriri, August 1986.

tion in fertility, while the other proximate determinants, affecting fecundity, are normally relatively invariant.

This permits the construction of a simple aggregate model for the measurement of the determinants of fertility. It depends upon the idea that the principal proximate determinants can be seen as acting to inhibit fertility. In their absence, fertility for a population would be at a theoretical maximum, essentially determined by the effect of the secondary proximate determinants. This level is called the total fecundity rate, which for most populations falls between 13 to 17 births per woman, with an average at 15.3 (Bongaarts and Potter 1983: 79, 120–2).

The influence of the principal proximate determinants can then be seen as reducing fertility below the total fecundity rate (TF). The combined inhibiting effect of all the principal proximate determinants reduces potential fertility to the population's actual or observed fertility level, the total fertility rate (TFR). If the fertility-inhibiting effect of marriage were to be removed, fertility would be equal to TM, the total marital fertility rate. Without contraception and induced abortion, fertility would be at the level of TN, the total natural marital fertility rate. Lastly, without any lactation or abstinence, fertility would increase to TF, the total fecundity rate. Such a model makes possible direct comparison of the relative importance of the different proximate determinants in contributing to the actual level of fertility in a population.

Before going on to apply the proximate determinants framework to fertility change in Rufiji, some reconsiderations of the standard model (as developed in Bongaarts and Potter's book) are necessary, because of factors determining the total fecundity rate. There is some evidence that the prevalence of disease factors—malaria and venereal disease—affecting spontaneous intrauterine mortality and sterility respectively, may be higher in the study area than the 'normal' levels assumed by Bongaarts and Potter. These factors are considered in turn.

Malaria

The main detailed evidence that malaria may have an unusually large effect on fecundity in coastal Tanzania comes from Bantje's (1987, 1988) work on the seasonality of births. Of particular relevance is the pattern of births at the mission-run maternity hospital in Ikwiriri. There is a seasonal peak of births at Ikwiriri during the dry, post-harvest season (July to October) corresponding to a conception peak during the period of early rains and agricultural labour (October to January). The seasonal trough for births occurs in the harvest and immediate post-rains season (March to May), corresponding to a conceptions trough post-harvest (June to September).

Bantje puts forward a number of possible causes for this seasonal pattern which, he argues, is real rather than an artefact of measurement error. These possibilities can be divided into direct behavioural influences on frequency of intercourse (especially for first births), and physiological factors acting either directly or indirectly through frequency of intercourse (Bantje 1988: 5–6).

He argues that the accumulated stress of a heavy workload, energy deficiency, anaemia, and malaria infection during the rainy season contributes to a reduced level of fecundity. The smallest number of births occurs when the second half of the gestation period coincides with the heavy agricultural labour of the early rains (November to January). Equally, births are highly (negatively) correlated with rainfall lagged four months before the time of conception, which, Bantje argues, shows the effect of malaria on spontaneous abortions in early pregnancy (Bantje 1988: 6). Lastly, both malaria and physical exhaustion are considered possibly to be acting through behavioural factors, morbidity inducing temporary sexual abstinence, especially during the immediate post-harvest and malarial season (June to July). All in all, Bantje attributes about half the seasonal variation to the effect of malaria and physical exhaustion on fecundity in general, and the other half to variations in pregnancy loss and sexual behaviour.

While all of these conclusions may be true, there is conflicting evidence from elsewhere. First, there is no epidemiological evidence to implicate malaria as a cause of sterility (Belsey 1976: 333). Secondly, while malaria has been observed to increase rates of spontaneous intrauterine mortality where it is epidemic, there is no clear association for populations where it is endemic (*Lancet* 1983) as it is in Rufiji. For these reasons, endemic malaria in sub-Saharan Africa has elsewhere been assessed as having an 'effect on fertility . . . negligible relative to the order of magnitude of expected levels of fetal loss' (Bongaarts *et al.* 1984: 526).

That the direct effect of malaria on pregnancy loss might not be so important is supported by the differential pattern of seasonality by birth order in Ikwiriri (Bantje 1988: 4). While the rate of malaria attacks peaks just after the rains (late May and June), conceptions for first births are above average at this time of year. Only with higher birth orders do conceptions at this period drop, suggesting either that other factors are involved or possibly that the effect of malaria is cumulative (United Republic of Tanzania 1973, iv: 144–5).

The other contradictory piece of evidence is that the seasonal pattern has shifted over time, with the conception trough coming slightly earlier in the year after 1980 than before. Bantje accounts for this by pointing to shifts in settlement and the decline of agriculture, but these factors implicate changes in workload and nutrition rather than in malarial infection *per se*. Only the overall reduction in seasonal variation over time may be partly attributable to the increased availability of malaria prophylaxis.

In summary, while the seasonal variations are very important, it seems likely that they are caused by variations in frequency of intercourse—either to do with gender relations (Bantje 1988: 5) or to do with morbidity—rather than directly by malaria and poor diet acting on pregnancy loss and fecundity.[3]

[3] See also Bongaarts and Potter (1983: 14–17).

Pathological sterility

Sterility or infertility, defined as the physiological incapacity to produce a live birth, runs at about 3 per cent in a normal population, this being the expected percentage of childless couples in a natural fertility regime where the wife is aged 20 (Bongaarts and Potter 1983: 41–2). A distinction is often made between primary sterility—childlessness—and the larger proportion of women who have one child but are unable to have another (secondary sterility). The two often have the same causes (Chatfield *et al.* 1970; Bongaarts *et al.* 1984: 527).

There is wide spread agreement that excess sterility in sub-Saharan Africa (which was and is quite extensive) is caused almost exclusively by gonorrhoea and post-abortal or post-partum infection (Chatfield *et al.* 1970; Belsey 1976: 320, 326–8, 333–4; Frank 1983: 138; Bongaarts *et al.* 1984: 527).

Primary sterility, in societies with natural or near-natural fertility, can be measured by the percentage of childless women at the end of their reproductive lives, i.e. ages 45–49. Secondary sterility can be measured similarly by the percentage of women aged 45–49 with one child. Given the 'normal' figure of 3 per cent, Tanzania's population clearly suffers from pathological primary infertility, the percentage childless being 17 per cent in 1948, 10.9 per cent in 1967, and 10.2 per cent in 1978 (Pearce 1986: 3–4). The problem in Coast Region is particularly severe, as was seen in Chapter 1.

Levels of childlessness in different countries, when compared with total fertility rates (TFRs), enable us to gauge the effects of pathological sterility on fecundity. Regressing TFRs on the percentage childless in eighteen sub-Saharan countries gives the result that infertility accounts for about 60 per cent of the variation in fertility (Frank 1983: 141), and 'that each 9 percentage point increment in the proportion of women 45–49 who are childless translates into a drop in total fertility of one live birth' (Bongaarts *et al.* 1984: 528).

Regressing reported parity for the age group 45–49 on percentage childless for the regions of Tanzania gives a very similar result (Pearce 1986: 19). On the basis of these regressions and the data in Table 1.8, the shortfalls in the TFR for Coast Region are: 1967–1.54; 1973–1.32; 1978–0.69. The estimate from the 1988 Census is, as noted in Chapter 1, unreliable.

It is worth noting that in the fitting of the regression for the regions of Tanzania, Coast Region is a low outlier, that is, total fertility is much lower than would be expected given the percentage childless. This will partly be due to the seasonal pattern of birth shortfalls discussed above. But it clearly also shows that other proximate determinants are inhibiting fertility more strongly than in other regions. It is to these principal determinants—marriage, contraception, and post-partum infecundability—that we now turn.

Contraception and abortion

As noted in Chapter 1, the parity progression ratio data for older women suggest the absence of strong parity-specific fertility control, which is usually associated with substantial contraceptive use. However, the use of contraception for spacing, rather than a stopping behaviour, is emerging as a distinctive African pattern (e.g. Bledsoe *et al.* 1994), so a closer examination of evidence on contraceptive prevalence is necessary.

Rufiji, and more generally Tanzania, had in 1985 a largely non-contracepting population, where 'contraception' is taken to mean modern methods of contraception. The sole supplier of contraceptives, both directly and through the Ministry of Health, was UMATI, the Tanzanian family-planning association.

The few sources of data on contraceptive use agree as to the order of magnitude of percentage take-up. A study of 773 women in 1979–81 in the regions of Kilimanjaro, Mara, and Morogoro—where much of the effort of UMATI has in the past been directed—shows contraceptive use rates of between 2.7 and 9.5 per cent, with an average of 6.58 per cent (Sembajwe 1984: tables 6 and 8). The Director of Programmes at UMATI himself estimated a take-up rate for Dar es Salaam of about 5 per cent (Rukonge 1985).

In Rufiji itself, data from the District Hospital[4] for January to July of 1985 show a total of 756 users of contraceptives, the vast majority being prescribed the pill. The number of married women aged 15–49 in the district recorded in the 1988 census was 23,292, so this represents a take-up rate for married women in the region of 3.25 per cent. Another source of data is part of the present study. One section of the birth and marriage history questionnaire administered in Ikwiriri between May and September 1986 contained questions about knowledge and use of modern contraception. Of 126 women aged 15–60, six (4.76 per cent) were currently using contraception.

The 1991–2 DHS recorded high levels of knowledge of modern methods (89.4 per cent) and of sources for obtaining those methods (79.7 per cent) for Coast Region. Nevertheless, recorded levels of current use of modern methods are very low, at 3.3 per cent of currently married women.

Marriage

Table 2.1 shows the percentage of women in 5-year age groups currently married for Coast Region in 1967, 1973, 1978, and 1988.

As can be seen from the table, a smaller proportion of women are getting married in the younger age groups—the converse of this being that the mean age at marriage is increasing. The singulate mean ages at marriage (SMAM) for Coast Region women are: 1967–16.48; 1973–18.57; 1978–19.10.

The SMAM measure is of some use in looking at an existing population as a synthetic cohort, although in populations with higher out-migration for married than unmarried women, as is likely here, it is biased downwards. However, it is less meaningful when *comparing* dates to estimate recent changes in ages at marriage. A more useful measure is derivable which attempts to project the future marriage behaviour of younger cohorts in the more recent censuses (Hajnal 1953: 120). However, as may be seen in Table 2.2, there is little difference between these measures and the simple SMAMs.

[4] I am indebted to Medical Assistant Seif Seleman Rashid for allowing me access to these figures.

Table 2.1. *Percentage of women married, by age group, Coast Region, 1967–1988*

Age group	1967 Census	1973 NDS	1978 Census	1988 Census
15–19	63.1	35.7	36.9	33.0
20–24	88.4	77.1	73.7	68.9
25–29	91.5	90.4	83.2	77.8
30–34	90.8	90.4	84.6	80.2
35–39	88.8	88.8	85.6	83.2
40–44	85.6	88.0	85.1	79.8
45–49	83.4	85.5	78.9	79.6

Sources: 1967—United Republic of Tanzania, *1967 Population Census*, iii; 1973—United Republic of Tanzania/Bureau of Statistics NDS, i: table 2,000; 1978—United Republic of Tanzania/Bureau of Statistics, *1978 Population Census*, vii: table 2; 1988—*1988 Population Census*, unpublished tables.

Table 2.2. *Singulate mean ages at marriage, 1973 and 1978 based on projected proportions single for ages over 35, Coast Region*

Year	SMAM		
1967		16.48	
1973	18.82[a]		18.61[b]
1978	18.88[a]		19.25[b]

[a] proportions projected on the assumption of constant marriage rates at higher ages.

[b] proportions projected on the assumption of uniform changes in marriage rates at higher ages.

Moreover, there are problems with applying this methodology, since the age pattern of proportions single does not show the qualities of a stable baseline. Nevertheless, they are the best available source on marriage ages.

The figures for the prevalence of marriage given in Table 2.1 show that although marriage is clearly the norm for women along the coast, it is not as universal as elsewhere in Tanzania. There are two factors at work. First, relatively high levels of divorce mean that in no age group does the percentage of women currently married much exceed 90 per cent. Secondly, there is a clear trend in the younger age groups towards later marriage, as reflected in the SMAM. Marital instability, together with sterility, was identified as a key

Table 2.3. *Proximate fertility determination, Rufiji District/Coast Region, 1967–1988*

Index	1967	1973	1978	1988
C_p	0.899	0.914	0.955	0.955
C_a	1.0	1.0	1.0	1.0
C_c	1.0	0.999[a]	0.981	0.971
C_m	0.829	0.707	0.700	0.676
TFR	4.9	5.1	5.3	5.476
Imputed C_i	0.43	0.516	0.528	0.571
Imputed av. birth interval (months)	46.5	38.7	37.8	35.0

[a] Assuming $u = 1.0\%$, $e = 0.90$. This figure for u is based on facts suggesting that while contraceptive services were available in villages from 1972, the 1973 data source dates from before the launch of integrated MCH/FP services in 1974.

Sources: 1967, 1978, 1988—Census volumes. 1973—*National Demographic Survey*, Bureau of Statistics, United republic of Tanzania.

element in low fertility on the coast by Tanner in his 1957–8 study of Pangani, in Tanga Region (Tanner 1959: 64–7). His data show an average of only 55–65 per cent of women aged over 20 currently in unions in the villages near Pangani.

The Proximate Determinants of Fertility in Rufiji/Coast Region, 1967–1978

With the information in the above sections, it is possible to construct a number of indices relating total fecundity to total fertility through the proximate determinants. This enables a comparison of the relative importance of each type of inhibiting effect on fertility (Table 2.3). The details of the calculations involved are given in Appendix 2.1.

The indicators in Table 2.3 are clearly provisional. They have been computed from data originally collected for other purposes and rely on a number of assumptions and simplifications. Nevertheless, they are a good first approximation to the kind of information needed for the study of the social control of fertility in coastal Tanzania. Each *C* index shows the depressing effect on fertility—the lower the index, the greater the effect.[5] In 1967, the most important proximate determinants were child-spacing (C_i), marriage (C_m) and

[5] As described in Appendix 2.1, normally the Bongaarts and Potter indices are estimated and then applied to the measured TFR to build up to a total fecundity rate of between 13 and 17. Here, however, because there is no detailed information on lactation, the relative weight of child-spacing variables is imputed, by assuming the Bongaarts and Potter 'standard' total fecundity rate of 15.3 and working downwards. This is justified on the rounds that we are interested in relative change over time, rather than absolute values.

pathological sterility (C_p). By 1978, the effect of sterility has lessened, although only modestly. Contraception (C_c), and probably abortion (C_a), have had negligible effect. The largest changes, however, have come with marriage, further depressing fertility through later first marriage for women, and probably with declining birth intervals, on average raising fertility over the period.

The levels of imputed birth intervals should not be taken too seriously, since the levels of some other factors, such as abortion, and sterility in 1988, are largely unknown. However, the imputed value of 35 months for 1988 is very close to the reported 34.6 months for the coastal zone in the 1991–2 TDHS. Similarly, the 46.5 months figure for 1967 is close to Ngallaba's estimate of around 48 months for women starting to bear children in 1940 (the centre of their fertility distribution would be about ten years later).

The analysis of these two chapters presents us with a set of problems for the next stage of explaining the history of fertility change in Rufiji. We know that fertility was probably static or slightly declining on the coast before 1950, and started rising thereafter, through to the 1980s. We also have some idea of how the proximate determinants of fertility changed from 1967 onwards. However, we know little about what happened before then. Specifically, we do not know exactly which change in proximate determinants was responsible for the shift in the fertility trend around 1950. Medical history and the pattern of parity progression ratios suggests that the decline of sterility may have been a primary factor. Certainly sterility was becoming increasingly less of a constraint on fertility by the 1970s. On the other hand, while sterility may have been the immediate cause of the beginning of the rise in fertility, this does not mean that other proximate determinants, especially those factors shown to be changing later on—marriage and birth intervals—were static before 1967. Clearly, at this stage, we need to move away from a narrowly demographic history to start to examine the institutional settings of marriage, divorce, post-partum abstinence, and breastfeeding, and the social and economic transformation which may have affected them.

Appendix 2.1: Calculation of the Bongaarts and Potter Indices

The procedures adopted here, and the principles underlying them, are fully explained in Bongaarts and Potter (1983). The usual procedure when using the model is to take the reported total fertility rate (TFR) and build up to a total fecundity rate of between thirteen and seventeen births per woman on the basis of information about each of the proximate determinants. Here, however, we have no detailed information on lactation, which will therefore have to be imputed. This can be done by taking the derived standard for total fecundity—15.3 births per woman—and working down towards the reported TFR.

The first stage is to take into account the inhibiting effects of pathological infertility. Using the estimate derived from the relationship between proportion childless at ages 45–49 and the total fertility rate, the shortfall for 1978 is 0.69. Thus we can adjust total fecundity downwards, to give an indicator of pathological sterility (C_p):

$$\frac{15.3 - 0.69}{15.3} = 0.955.$$

The original Bongaarts and Potter 15.3 figure for total fecundity is thus reduced for 1978 down to

$$15.3 \times 0.955 = 14.61.$$

The next step is to take contraception and abortion into account. In the absence of any quantitative information about abortion, the abortion index, C_a, may be taken as 1.0. C_c, the contraceptive index, is given by the expression;

$$C_c = 1 - 1.08 \times u \times e,$$

where u = the proportion currently using contraception among married women of reproductive age, and e = the average use-effectiveness of contraception (Bongaarts and Potter 1983: 82–4). On the basis of the discussion above, u is taken to be about 2 per cent for 1978, while e is taken to be 0.90.[6] C_c is therefore:

$$1 - 1.08 \times 0.02 \times 0.9 = 0.981.$$

This means that total fecundity net of contraception and abortion is given by:

$$14.61 \times 0.981 = 14.33.$$

The next stage in the calculation is to bring in the effects of marriage. C_m, the marriage index, is calculated as the weighted sum of the proportion of women in each age group who are married, the weights being the age-specific marital fertility rates (Bongaarts and Potter 1983: 81–2). For 1978 this is 0.6998, which means that the effect of marriage:

$$14.33 \times 0.6998 = 10.03.$$

The difference between this figure and the reported total fertility rate is now entirely due to the effects of post-partum infecundability. The index of post-partum infecundability is given by the expression:

$$C_i = \frac{20}{18.5 + i},$$

[6] This is the figure used by Bongaarts and Potter for the pill, which is the most widely prescribed type of contraceptive in Rufiji.

where i is the length of the infecundable period, and $i + 18.5$ is the birth interval (Bongaarts and Potter 1983: 86–7). C_i is the ratio of the recorded TFR to 10.03, i.e.

$$5.3/10.03 = 0.528.$$

Substituting this value for C_i in the above expression gives us an estimate of the birth interval:

$$i + 18.5 = \frac{20}{0.528} = 37.8.$$

The infecundable period is $37.8 - 18.5 = 19.3$ months.

We can now provide a summary comparison of the indices for 1978:

C_p (pathological sterility) = 0.955,
C_a (abortion) = 1.0,
C_c (contraception) = 0.981,
C_m (marriage) = 0.6998,
C_i (postpartum infecundability) = 0.528,
i (length of infecundable period) = 19.3 months,
$i + 18.5$ (birth interval) = 37.8 months.

The indices for 1967, 1973, and 1988 were derived in an identical fashion.

3 The Historical Roots of a Fertility Regime

The picture of human reproduction in Rufiji drawn together from various sources and presented in the previous two chapters remains hazy. There is much that we do not know. Nevertheless, the outlines of a particular fertility regime are discernible: early and universal marriage for women, long birth intervals, high sterility, and high levels of marital instability. There are also indications of patterns over time: demographic crisis in the early colonial years, followed by stagnant fertility and mortality up to the 1950s. In the post-Second World War years fertility begins to rise, probably because of falls in sterility and a shortening of the birth interval, but counteracted by a rise in age at first marriage for women.

How are such patterns related to the social and economic history of Rufiji? What are the origins of the fertility regime and why has it changed? Has it indeed been transformed? The analysis of the proximate determinants of fertility in Chapter 2 provides a preliminary step in approaching these questions. However, without a wider understanding of the social and economic institutions within which these determinants were set, our answers will precisely remain preliminary. The challenge here is to investigate the social and economic structure of reproductive relations, and determinants of reproductive change, in a way which does not reduce fertility to a functional corollary of the outcome of social or economic forces.

The approach taken in the following two chapters is to start with two sets of relations—those to do with the formation of marriage as a reproductive union, and those between husband and wife within marriage—and work outwards to the institutions of political, spatial, and economic organization in Rufiji. Applying such a process to the past inevitably links arguments to sources. For example, the pattern of early and near-universal marriage for women, common for Africa, is usually associated with a degree of polygyny (Lesthaeghe *et al.* 1989). It has also been taken to reflect a desire on the part of men to capture the productive and reproductive potential of women as bearers of children and agricultural workers (Lesthaeghe 1980, 1989*b*). While these elements were present in Rufiji, and indeed are evident in the issues of conjugal conflict and marital instability discussed below, the treatment below focuses on the historical roots of marriage formation as basically a political process, a treatment which arises out of the sources. The analysis offers interpretations which are non-deterministic, but which remain partial.

Origins and History in Rufiji

This chapter attempts to create a history of Rufiji. Two related dangers face any such attempt. One concerns the identification of an 'original' society, a timeless pre-colonial local world. The other is the attempt to identify the 'true' characteristics of such a society, to label it, for example, 'matrilineal' or 'patrilineal'. To avoid these dangers it is necessary to interpret all sources as a comment on a changing society, and to recognize how any one set of evidence supports different interpretations.

It becomes possible to trace the currents of change by the mid-nineteenth century, with the growth of centres of trade around the delta and along the river and southern Ungindo trade routes, with links to the larger centres at Zanzibar and Kilwa. Social and economic transformation was further and brutally accelerated by the German forced-labour cotton schemes, response to the MajiMaji uprising, colonial agricultural and commercial policy, usury and extraction by merchant capital, and the attempts at Indirect Rule.

This process was continuous, if uneven. Rufiji society never existed in isolation, and indeed was continually renewed and changed by waves of migration from the south and west, so it would be misleading to talk of an 'original' form of organization in the west and hills, and a 'new' form in the delta towns and later river settlements. Firstly, there is evidence that, from the rise of the Shirazi dynasty in about AD 1200, the Rufiji delta and fertile flood basin served a succession of coastal entrepôts—Kilwa, Mafia, and Zanzibar—as a hinterland rich in both food and products for export (Freeman-Grenville 1965: 50; Kjekshus 1977: 30; Oliver 1977: 184, 186). Secondly, according to oral histories collected by colonial officers, an important part of the accounts of the southern Rufiji societies is provenance in groups of migrants, marginalized or expelled, from the coast (Kilwa) and the interior (Uhehe) (TNA 61/3/VI/D; Provincial Commissioner's Report, Eastern Province, 1931; RH, 'Tribal Histories'). Later migrations brought other groups from the south and west, leading to a mixing of identifications—Ngindo, Pogoro, Makonde, etc.—especially in the upstream areas.

Thus, although the Rufiji peoples do not appear in any of the standard English or German ethnographies, they fall geographically and culturally at the interstices of two or possibly three major identified systems (Biedelman 1967; Prins 1967; Wembah-Rashid 1975), and so some comparisons and extrapolations are possible. One assertion is based on the group of matrilineal societies ranging through eastern Tanzania from the area east of Morogoro to the south beyond the Ruvuma. On the basis of this 'matrilineal belt', and the fact that it has been argued that the Rufiji valley and southern hills are peopled essentially by migrants from this area, an original state of matrilineality has been claimed for the people of Rufiji (Swantz, 1985: 24).[1] On the other hand, young

[1] This has also been argued for other coastal peoples e.g. the Wazaramo (Swantz, 1970: 111), the people of Mafia (Caplan 1982).

men in Rufiji in the 1980s were adamant that their society and always been patrilineal.

For our purposes, however, neither ethnicity nor the identification of a system as matri- or patri-lineal is that important. The accuracy of detail in colonial accounts of 'tribal histories' has been questioned (Rufiji District Books, 'Notes by R. V. Hartnoll'), and their relevance for the identity of the migrants once they had arrived must also be in doubt. It is likely that many people living in Rufiji used ethnic and cultural identity quite instrumentally to meet specific social or political ends. At one level, this sometimes meant assimilation into a clan, often for the purposes of gaining rights to land. Since land rights were held by recognized local lineages, for incoming groups this frequently meant marrying into an existing clan, making such marriages effectively uxorilocal. Equally, ethnic identity in Rufiji, at least as it has come to be maintained, remains a malleable category. It can be claimed on a spectrum of genealogical size, from narrowly defined clan groups (*ukoo*) (Beardall 1881: 642–4), to the 'tribal' identities of Ndengereko, Matumbi, etc., and ultimately at the wider level of the whole Rufiji, usually in contradistinction to other parts of the coast. This is reflected in language names. There are three main languages spoken in the district, other than Kiswahili: Kindengereko, Kirufiji, and Kimatumbi. However, they are closely related and mutually intelligible, and outsiders often refer to the language block, as well as the people, simply as 'Rufiji'. For our purposes here, the smaller groups are so similar in language, culture, and political structure that broad categorization is sufficient.

With respect to the issue of the line of descent (i.e. through the female or male line), as will emerge below, while nominal patriliny is now long-standing in Rufiji, this does not necessarily mean much in terms of political, economic, or residential organization. 'Rules' were often broken and reinterpreted, so that accounts of actual relationships seem more useful than discussion about origins.

Marriage, Space, and Politics

An important feature of the fertility regime in Rufiji has been early and universal marriage for women. Part of the reason for this must be, as elsewhere in sub-Saharan Africa, the value accorded to the productive and reproductive powers of women, and the desire on the part of men to control those powers. However, as becomes clear in the discussion of marital instability below, making a marriage did not mean that it would last, and conjugal relations in Rufiji have often been characterized by conflict. The dynamics of men appropriating the labour of women through marriage is therefore much more traceable through relations within unions than in union formation. At the same time, the sources on early Rufiji history point us in a different direction, seeing marriage formation bound up with political and geographical organization. In late precolonial Rufiji, settlement consisted largely of scattered hamlets, made up of small numbers of households related by kinship. Marriages were links between the hamlets, and played key roles in survival during periods of crisis.

It is clear from the direct accounts of travellers and oral historians that precolonial Rufiji was acephalous, with an essentially egalitarian political ideology.[2] A common pattern of political and social organization emerges, both for the 'matrilineal' societies such as Mwera and Kwere, and the 'patrilineal' ones such as Ngindo and Hehe (MaijiMaji Research Project nos. 7/68/2/1/ and 7/68/2/3/5; RH, 'Tribal Histories of Wamatumbi and Wakichi'; Cross-Upcott 1956; Vuorella 1986). A basic political and residential unit was what Cross-Upcott called the 'lineage cell', i.e. 'a loose cluster of up to a dozen agnates along with their families and dependants' (Cross-Upcott 1956: 26). At a larger scale, beyond this local lineage was a clan whose heads in southern Rufiji frequently adopted the title of *Mpindo*, and who sometimes became the focus of Indirect Rule policies (RH, 'Tribal Histories').

But the point was that such leaders or elders acted mostly as arbitrators for peace in larger-scale disputes: 'They were in no sense chiefs, or even petty headmen, so small was their scope and so limited their function' (Cross-Upcott 1956: 112).[3] A recollection of the pre-MajiMaji Wamwera stresses this purely advisory or negotiating role of extra-cell leaders:

> Wamwera hawakuwa na mpango wowote wa ukubwa kwa kabila . . . kila ukoo ulijikusanya pamoja na kukaa. Mzee zaidi wa mwenye jina aliheshimiwa kama kiongozi wao, lakini hawakuwa na madaraka kwa mtu wowote, ila aliweza kukusanya wazee wenziwe na kufanya nao shauri lolote la maana. Wakishauriana, wanakubali, lakini hakuweza kulazimisha au kuadhibu
>
> (The Wamwera didn't have any plan at all at the scale of tribe . . . each clan collected itself together and settled. The elder of the name was respected as their leader, but he had no responsibility for anyone, except he could gather his elders and conduct with them any matter of importance. If they consulted together, they agreed, but he [the leader] could not force or punish). (MajiMaji Research Project No. 7/68/2/1)

Within the lineage cell, or lineage hamlet, descent principles to some extent determined residence, but there were often exceptions, and patriliny certainly did not make uterine kin unimportant (Cross-Upcott 1956: 26). Cross-Upcott writes:

> The [patri-]lineage cell is the typical residential unit; but not to the exclusion of all other types or combinations. One finds a considerable minority of cases where uterine kin or affines form appendages to agnatic nuclei, mostly in the shapes of suitors who have stayed on as uxorilocal husbands, their issue, as uterine relatives of the old inhabitants, belonging there permanently. There is also a sprinkling of elderly ailing or needy persons who have become satellites of their more robust, but not necessary agnatic, kinsmen. (Cross-Upcott 1956: 111)

[2] This is the standard view of the nature of political organization in the whole southern hinterland: see Gray (1976: 507). Certainly, when Beardall made his visit to Rufiji in 1885, the political jurisdiction of the 'chiefs' whom he encountered did not even fully hold within the hamlets which formed their lineage groups, let alone beyond. At this stage, the society away from the trading centres was decentralized (Beardall 1881: 647). See also Iliffe (1979: 21–2).

[3] See also MajiMaji Research Project No. 7/68/2/1.

The local lineage cells were bound together, both internally and externally, by marriage ties:

> Ngindo society, its agnatic cells too minute and flabby to form a hard structure, resembles a non-vertebrate creature, possessing a hard shell. That shell is kinship. Ngindo for the most part seek their spouses away from the home settlement. The result is a complex web of kinship flung right across Ngindoland. (Cross-Upcott 1956: 119)

Another observer describes the people of Rufiji as all 'belonging to one big endogamous ring' (RH, 'Notes by R. V. Hartnoll').

According to Vuorella, who describes similar 'domestic communities' of Wakwere near Morogoro, this form of social organization (which she sees as bound up with matrilineality) was related to the system of land-use which put a premium on the mobility of labour, and hence the need for friendly relationships over a wide area. For the matrilineal Wakwere, this was facilitated through the distribution of related men by uxorilocal marriage:

> [M]atrilineal social organisation creates friendly ties of kinship and cooperation between a wider group of men and domestic communities than in those societies where males, united by strong fraternal interest groups, are concentrated in one locality. (Vuorella 1986: 19)

I would argue that even in nominally patrilineal societies of 'lineage cell' organization—and we have seen that many of them were effectively partially bilineal—strong links with affinal kin can play the same role of sharing resources in times of local famine, illness, or political crisis.

In Rufiji this role was particularly important in view of variation in the spatial organization of settlement, which in the late nineteenth century appears to have been influenced by political, agricultural, and environmental factors. Apart from the requirements of kinship and marriage, as outlined above, there was a need to balance protection from wild animals, and in the valley from floods, against the demands of production in terms of access to good-quality land. What emerged was a geographically differentiated pattern.

In the hill areas, the segmented lineage hamlet was a small, highly mobile unit, allowing shifting cultivation. In the upstream area, the unstable flooding regime, slave raids, and war with the Ngoni also encouraged small mobile settlements (Bantje 1979: 32). Settlement further downstream was either in ribbon-like villages strung out along the levees, or even in nucleated villages, such as those observed by Elton in the 1870s (ibid.). These more concentrated patterns were reinforced and spread by German colonial policy, in which villages were created along the roads, improving access (TNA 1733/17/11/10).

The ribbon pattern reflected the primacy of the river in communications and trade, and gave some protection from flooding and wild animals. But this protection was limited, and Matzke has argued that, by blocking access to the river for animals, the settlement pattern actually increased the game–human contact (Bantje 1979: 33).

It is clear that the excess variation in the ecological setting of the Rufiji strongly militated for such links, and they remain important today.[4] But equally clearly, some groups failed in this strategy, and both at times of wider crisis (e.g. large-scale famine) and with the progressive commoditisation and monetization of relationships, mutual security became exchange. Thus there are accounts of the selling of children for food in the German period,[5] and later of bartering between refugees from famine in the valley and people in the hills (TNA 61/3/XIII/D).

If marriage was the 'shell' knitting together lineage hamlets where the political influence of hamlet heads was nominal and their rights merely 'paternal' (RH, 'Tribal Histories'), it was also a key political instrument for a society in which civil power was synonymous with domestic power. For marriages mattered: they would be judged partially by their contribution to the construction of the 'shell', and hence were likely to be controlled by agnatic kin. Further, it was clearly easier to control marriages between hamlets than within hamlets. Control of marriage, through the organization of marriage payments and directly through influence over propsective bride and groom, was therefore a central issue:

> Marriage is the bridge between the multitudinous Ngindo social units. The latter can dispense with all other permanent commitments, but by marriage alone can they perpetuate themselves. Therefore by hook or by crook, spouses must be found. When found they must be held
>
> A stable link should be forged when the metal is still pliable. So groups try to secure marriage partners in advance, and to indoctrinate them thoroughly. (Cross-Upcott 1956: 257)

Gender, Economy, and Rite

The setting of marriage formation in late nineteenth century Rufiji was political and spatial organization. Once marriages were formed, however, subsequent relations between husband and wife, encompassing sexual abstinence, conflict, separation, and divorce, were closely bound up with the roles of men and women in agricultural production. Gender relations consisted of sets of expectations and more or less explicit conflict over the breaking of roles. Expectations of behaviour in sexual and productive arenas were constantly linked through metaphor and symbol in the practice and cosmological language of rites, especially puberty rites. Gender relations of production and conjugal relations were thus embedded in each other.

[4] Thus, when asked if kin were important for mutual aid, a young man living some distance from his area of origin replied that the more important aspect was the spread of connections: 'If you arrive somewhere as a stranger, but you can find kin, you will be all right' (interview with Moshi Mokea 26.2.1986). Young men in Mng'aru also stressed the importance of maintaining the communication of information through the *ukoo* (interviews with Moshi Mokea and Koba Ngurupi, 11.3.1986).

[5] Interview with Shabani Mpyomi, 19.4.1986; RH, i (1937).

A gendered economy

The accounts of early travellers and of ethnographers working in nearby areas provide some basis for reconstructing the conditions of production, but there are severe limitations to the backward projection involved. Elton, passing through the flood plain in 1874, noted the participation of men, women, and children in agriculture.[6] Cross-Upcott worked much later in Ungindo, in the far south-west of the district, before the creation of the Selous game reserve. Although he was describing a system of land-use and labour in the 1950s, it was in an area with relatively little intensive contact with either administration or markets. Labour migration appeared to have been the major innovation in the local economy. As elsewhere over most of the hill areas, shifting cultivation was practised: while land was freely available, definite individual rights (for both men and women) were held over cleared and planted fields (Cross-Upcott 1956: 40–2). He also describes a gender division of labour with women concentrating on food-processing, brewing, water and wood collection; men on food-gathering, hunting, bee-keeping, clearing of fields and crafts; and both on agriculture (ibid. 75–6).

A deeper understanding of the moral obligations of gender in production can be gained by delving into the roots of the major political crisis of the early colonial period—the MajiMaji war. The MajiMaji rebellion originated south of Rufiji in July 1905, and spread right across southern Tanzania before it was finally defeated with great brutality in 1907 (Iliffe 1967, 1969). Two points about MajiMaji are relevant. First, that the reason for the original outbreak of rebellion—forced labour on cotton schemes—is only properly and fully understood by consideration of the domestic economy and gender divisions of labour, and hence illuminates those factors. Second, that the main factor in the spread of rebellion—the unifying ideology of MajiMaji—derived its form and symbolism from part of a body of ritual practice which both defined gender identity and strengthened gender solidarity.

This is not an argument that MajiMaji was wholly about crises of a domestic nature: both Gwassa and Iliffe remind us that it was, especially after the initial stage, a nationalist war of independence where the key issue became the possibility of political and military unity among the peoples of southern Tanzania (MajiMaji Research Project No. 7/68/1/3/15; Iliffe 1967: 495; 1969: 7; Gwassa 1972: 202). But the imposition of colonial extraction only sparked protest and uprising, and the uprising only became mass rebellion because of factors deeply rooted in what is often referred to as the 'domestic sphere'.[7]

The setting for the MajiMaji rebellion was German colonial rule, with taxation, harsh punishment for default, forced labour in road construction, and substantial misrule on the part of the colonial state's agents (Iliffe 1969: 21). But these were felt all over the country, and the immediate cause of MajiMaji was more specific to the southern coastal area.

[6] RH, 'Extracts from Elton'.

[7] For the importance of explaining why MajiMaji occurred when and where it did see Iliffe (1969: 21).

This was a cotton-growing scheme, introduced by Governor Götzen and financed by a group of German textile manufacturers under pressure from the US cotton-suppliers' cartel. The scheme was imposed under a brutal regime of beatings, and there were effectively no returns to labour. In addition, the entire process of production was completely subsumed under state control: the cotton plots were laid out by the headman's house, often some distance from the labourers' homes; each person had to work a specified number of days; inputs (i.e. seeds), cultivation, and marketing were overseen by a European-controlled committee; and the division of proceeds, even in theory, gave only one-third to the labourers, the rest going to headmen and to the committee (Iliffe 1967: 497–8).

The importance of this for existing agricultural processes was noted both at the time, and in subsequent accounts. Originally, only adult men were supposed to be conscripted, but in their absence from a house, or as they began to refuse, women and children were drafted in (Gwassa and Iliffe 1967; Iliffe 1967: 498–9). To begin to see exactly how the inflexible demands of the cotton scheme distorted the household-level economy, a longer quote from a Kipatimu resident is illuminating:

> [P]eople suffered much from the cotton, which took three months [to ripen] and was picked in the fourth. Now digging and planting were in the months of Ntandatu and Nchimbi and this was the time of very many wild pigs in this country. If you left the chasing of the pigs to the woman she could not manage well at night. In addition [the pigs] are very stubborn at that period and will not move even if you go within very close range. Only very few women can assist their husbands at night and these are the ones with very strong hearts. There were just as many birds, and if you did not have children it was necessary to help your wife to drive away the birds, while at the same time you cleared a piece of land for the second maize crop, because your wife would not have time. And during this very period they still wanted you to leave your home and go to . . . work on the *jumbe*'s plantation. This was why people became furious and angry. (*Mzee* Ndundule Mangaya, quoted in Gwassa and Iliffe 1967: 4)

The Germans were aware that women in Rufiji, and indeed in southern Tanzania generally, played a central role in agricultural production. They may have further inferred that they could therefore remove men from farming in order to extract surplus from the system, and, further, that women's agriculture was subsumed under their husbands' control.

However, what the above quote shows quite clearly is not only that the hill-farming systems involved a gender-specific division of tasks (with both male and female labour going into the cultivation of a particular crop), but also that the cotton scheme threatened what was essentially a system of reciprocal rights and duties in agriculture. The men hated the cotton scheme not only because it was brutally imposed and completely unremunerative, but also because its inflexible schedule, clashing with existing crop timetables, made them default on their gender-specific responsibilities in production. And these responsibilities were in turn part of the basis for their political rights to be household heads in a system with little political power above the domestic level, as described above. For these reasons, as well as directly through their own conscription, the cotton scheme affected women too, so that women came to play an important part in the preparations for the uprising. Indeed, when it came to the day, one of the three elders who uprooted cotton in late July 1905, marking the start of the rebellion, was a female *mganga*, Nantabila Naupunda (Gwassa 1972: 214).

A common language

One of the key points about MajiMaji was that the response to agricultural oppression very quickly took on a cosmological dimension. The main factor in the spread of rebellion—the unifying ideology of MajiMaji—derived its form and symbolism from ritual practice primarily addressed to problems of cultivation and family conflicts. The ideology which enabled a local uprising to spread across ethnic divisions, and be sustained for three years derived its force from a cosmology which not only specified hierarchical relationships between God, spirits such as Bokero, ancestors, and the living, but also located humankind in relation to the natural world.[8]

The *maji* (water) of the movement was not only thought to protect men from bullets, but also played the role of a 'general agricultural panacea', administered by women (Gwassa and Iliffe 1967: 10; Gwassa 1972: 206). *Maji*, or 'water' in the sense of water transformed into *dawa* or medicine, is still the central instrument of potency in protection against witchcraft in Rufiji.

The connection between the cosmology of southern coastal Tanzanian societies around the turn of the century and the gendered moral economy of cultivation is not visible solely through the exigencies of MajiMaji. The social construction and regulation of mutual responsibilities between men and women in general occurred largely through rites which were based on that cosmology. Thus teachings were made about both economic and sexual roles within the context of an overall account of relations between men, women, and the natural world.

This argument cannot rest on direct contemporary nineteenth-century evidence, since there is none. However, detailed accounts of initiation rites for both men and women along the coast suggest that such practices are long-standing (Swantz 1970; Caplan 1976; Strobel 1979). For instance, aspects of current Rufiji ceremony—such as the figure of *mkungwi*, an instructor of the girl who imparts knowledge about sex and menstruation, so that this role is not taken by the girl's mother—is found also in Mombasa as early as the late nineteenth century (Strobel 1979). The *mwali* rites of Rufiji are part of a larger East and Central African complex of puberty initiation institutions. The symbolic interpretation of these rites has always invoked the centrality of cosmology (Biedelman 1967; Turner 1967; Swantz 1970; Brain 1978).

An important element to these rites is the way in which sexuality is embedded in social and economic relations. In girls' puberty rites (*unyago*) on Mafia, for example, a girl is allotted a sexual instructress (*mkungwi*) who advises her

[8] MajiMaji Research Project 1/68/2/1; Gwassa 1972: 204–6. Bokero was the spirit or divinity from whose shrine the magical *maji* was obtained.

on menstruation and on sexual relations with her future husband (Caplan 1976). At the same time, *unyago* also teaches the adolescent about a wide range of appropriate behaviour and about the importance of kinship and agricultural work (ibid. 23, 27).[9] Similar rites are carried out at circumcision for boys.

Sexuality dominates the *unyago*. In Caplan's interpretation it pervades the other teachings, linked through symbolism both to farming and to cognatic kinship. The construction of female sexuality is presented in an ambiguous way. On the one hand, sex is presented as 'pleasurable for its own sake—not just in order to beget children' (Caplan 1976: 27) and women are expected to have extramarital affairs. On the other hand, women are taught that sexuality is one of their most powerful levers, both inside and outside of marriage (ibid. 28). This draws sexuality into an exchange relationship between men and women, not only for gifts, but also as part of their general relationships encompassing household management, work, relations with kin, and so on.

These institutions are of particular importance when trying to understand a long period of abstinence from sexual intercourse after birth, associated with long birth intervals. Analyses of abstinence have typically correlated a long post-partum 'taboo' with a certain type of social structure, involving polygyny and gerontocratic control (Saucier 1972; Schoenmaeckers *et al.* 1981; Lesthaeghe and Eelens 1989). Here, however, I am interested primarily in tracing the way in which abstinence behaviour was taught, learned, and changed.

In many cases, it appears that abstinence is motivated through the idiom of pollution: in Yorubaland, for example, the danger is that sperm will 'poison' the breast milk, and so endanger the child (Orubuloye 1981: 225; Caldwell and Caldwell 1981: 81). In the case of coastal Tanzania, therefore, given a rich cosmology linking human action and vulnerability to the natural and supernatural world, and a set of rites in which the teaching of sexuality predominates, we would expect to find a prominent role for the teaching of post-partum sexual abstinence. In fact, at least in recent rite, it is conspicuous by its absence. In Mafia, teaching about abstinence is not part of *unyago*.[10] In Marja-Liisa Swantz's voluminous work on symbol and rite in Zaramo society (1985), there is no mention of abstinence during breastfeeding. Sexual abstinence rules (although they are in any case weak, and counteracted by medicines) apply to pollution associated with menstrual blood, to the later stages of pregnancy, and to the immediate heat of childbirth (Swantz 1986: 264, 322–32).

Abstinence thus appears to be a more practical affair, often managed initially by the woman staying with her mother's kin for a period after giving birth. In Rufiji, current ideas about abstinence do not really relate to sexual

[9] The agricultural idiom has persisted. It is interesting to note that the adopted Kiswahili phrase for family planning is *uzazi wa majira*, which translates literally as parenthood according to the seasons. It is taken to refer to the spacing of births rather than their overall limitation. At least since MajiMaji, human fertility and agricultural fertility have been analogous.

[10] Pat Caplan, personal communication.

avoidance, but to pregnancy and child development.[11] Having another child should not be considered until a child 'has got his health' (*mpaka amepata afya yake*). However, a child can be weaned, even abruptly, if she or he is 'grown up' enough (*amekuwa*). Women who do become pregnant while breastfeeding will wean the child immediately.

There are two possible interpretations of this situation. One is that while previously, some prohibition on sexual intercourse during breastfeeding existed, backed by cosmological force, it has lost much of its power. Indeed, a shift over time in the nature of puberty rites is noted by some observers. Both Strobel and Swantz, who deal explicitly with developments in coastal initiation rites, point to a narrowing of the previously multivalent symbolism, and a reduction in the intensity and moral scope of the knowledge imparted (Swantz 1970: 225; Strobel 1979: 206–9). What was previously an experience of transformation and incorporation into an adult, gender-specific cosmology has become a way of teaching proper manners and behaviour.

Of course, it has always been possible to analyse initiation rites at several levels, at the social as well as the symbolic. But on this interpretation it is the loss of the cosmological dimension which significantly reduces the power of sanctions, and hence leads to non-observance. It is easier to break social rules, especially if one can get away with it, than to go against injunctions based on cosmological fear (where there is no possibility of hiding behaviour).[12]

The historical puzzle for this view is to understand why such a shift might have occurred; how it may be linked to forces which threatened the cosmology from without, such as Islam, or from within, such as a breakdown in the system of mutual rights and responsibilities of men and women in both agriculture and marriage.

The second interpretation is more straightforward. This is that there was no 'taboo', now eroded, but rather that abstinence has been of the form described above, i.e. avoiding pregnancy while breastfeeding. In these circumstances, resumption and frequency of sexual intercourse is a more pragmatic and personal issue between husband and wife, embedded in the construction of sexuality and associated conjugal relations of household and farm management. The historical issue here is tracing the implications for child spacing through changing patterns of economic and sexual pressure on women.

It is my view that the second interpretation is more plausible, mainly because of the striking absence of teaching of abstinence in accounts of the *unyago*.

[11] I have argued elsewhere Lockwood (1995) that anthropological evidence from a wide range of sources supports a view that 'post-partum abstinence' collapses a number of distinct practices together. In some African societies, abstinence is related to the polluted status of the mother after childbirth; in others to lactation; in yet others (as in Rufiji) it is pregnancy rather than sex which is to be avoided during breastfeeding, or until specific markers of child development have been attained.

[12] It is worth noting that when the decline of child spacing in Tanzania is discussed in the press now, it is entirely within the idiom of morality and decency.

4 Twentieth-century Transformations

The political, spatial, and economic organization of Rufiji underwent considerable change over the twentieth century, in ways which had ramifications for reproductive relations. The evidence points to a rather complex web of interrelating factors leading to three broad reproductive outcomes. Firstly, struggles between husbands and wives over control of labour, and later of rice, contributed to general marital instability, accommodated by the conception of marriage within Islam. Second, the relative economic positions of men and women were transformed by male out-migration, a diversification of the male economy, and villagization. New kinds of vulnerability for women, together with an increasingly antagonistic conjugal relationship, led to more pressure on women to resume sexual intercourse earlier, leading to shorter birth intervals. Third, under the influence of Islam and villagization, the existing basis of marriage, combining lineage power with political and spatial organization, became increasingly to do with relationships between individuals, and the resources of the bridegroom, which in turn were often dependent on migration.

Each of these arguments is elaborated in the next chapter. However, in order to understand each element, a broad sketch of twentieth-century transformations of Rufiji life is necessary. This encompasses the creation of a colonial economy and administration, the rise of Islam, post-war migration to Dar es Salaam, the diversification of the male economy, and villagization.

The Creation of a Colonial Economy

As we have seen, certain areas of Rufiji—particularly the delta and lower floodplain—had experienced at least one hundred years of contact with external markets, money, and merchant capital before the advent of German colonial invasion.[1] However, the effect on the economy up to this point was limited in two ways. First, geographically, because the spread of commodity production and consumption was very limited (RH, 'Extracts from Elton'; Iliffe 1979: 133); and, second, because commodity relations did not affect production directly, but only indirectly through trade. Both limitations were due to the

[1] Probably many more: see Sheriff (1987: 8).

political weakness of the Zanzibari traders and the military weakness of the Zanzibari state (Iliffe 1979: 46–9; Sheriff 1987: 2–4).

These limits become evident with the transition to colonial rule. With a number of measures, the colonial state intensified the need for commodity production. Production became more subsumed under direct state control. Merchants also gained more power as cycles of economic reproduction came to include more and more commodities.

A major initial instrument of transformation was taxation. Following the creation of German East Africa as a colony in early 1885, the first 'hut tax' ordinance came in 1897, and the first taxes were levied in 1898 (*Handbook of German East Africa* 1916: 19; Iliffe 1969: 160). For the first two or three years, payment in kind was accepted, and was apparently perceived as not particularly onerous. But after this honeymoon period, with a switch to payment in cash and oppressive penalties for default, taxation become a heavy burden. Indeed, monetary taxation in Rufiji was only fully imposed on the population by means of subjugation through military campaigns.[2]

Colonial taxes seem to have been designed to have various roles in different divisions of the colonial economy. In Rufiji, MajiMaji had made it clear that plantation and corvée labour was largely unworkable, and peasant commodity production was encouraged instead, tax being one spur (TNA 1733/5; TNA 1733/17/1/10; TNA 61/3/VI/D). However, another result was the stimulation of migration, mostly to Dar es Salaam, which by the 1930s was growing slowly but steadily. This was true especially in years of crop failure (TNA 1733/18: 105; RH, 'Notes on Census').

As Walter Rodney and John Iliffe have pointed out, the economic role of the Tanganyikan colony was set in the first decade of the twentieth century with the decision to favour peasant agriculture at the expense of settler agriculture (Iliffe 1969; Rodney 1983: 14). This was partly due to the experience of MajiMaji as a response to forced and supervised cotton cultivation. After 1907 this different approach was tried, and seed was distributed for the cultivation of cotton as a true *Volkskultur*. Both acreages and incomes grew rapidly. Indeed, by 1914, Rufiji was emerging as a major export crop area with most cultivation being on smallholdings, although there were some small plantations established between 1907 and 1910 (Telford 1929: 12; Iliffe 1969; Rodney 1983). The encouragement and acceptance of cotton cultivation in this manner was in part a response to the high world price up to and including the First World War.

The 1920s saw the post-war recovery of the Rufiji economy, with rice and cotton as mainstays. Cotton production had been systematized by the state, with both the supply of inputs (seeds) and the buying of the crop organized or overseen by the administration. For the district officers, this was an optimistic period, with attempts at extending cotton cultivation, the introduction of sesame as a hill cash-crop, and general enthusiasm for the agricultural potential of the district (TNA 1733/1, 5; TNA 1733/18: 105).

[2] *MajiMaji Research Project Collected Papers*, nos. 7/68/1/3/15, 7/68/2/3/1, 7/68/2/3/1, 7/68/1/3/15; Iliffe (1979: 133).

However, this early agricultural promise was never realized. Within the colonial economy of Tanganyika, Rufiji was only briefly an important export crop-producing area, and it was never a major labour reserve for the north-eastern sisal estates. Rather, it came to play the role of an 'intermediate' region, supplying food and some seasonal labour migration to the coastal towns (Iliffe 1979: 274).

From 1929, the whole colonial economy was affected by the world Depression, and commodity prices, including that of cotton, tumbled (Coulson 1982: 48). But for Rufiji, the crash came at the end of three decades of not so much underdevelopment as non-development. Farming and communications were heavily undercapitalized, and productivity relatively low. The whole period of the early 1930s was one of crisis, where the squeeze on reproduction—low producer prices, high taxes, and high consumer prices, augmented by vulnerability to drought and flooding—almost led to the breakdown of the system, as the 1931 District Report makes clear: 'The standard of living of the Rufiji native agriculturalist is such that even a slight fall in prices affects him, reducing his margin of profit to a degree that renders him unable to meet the normal demands of government' (TNA 61/3/VI/D).

Cotton, its price stagnant, became unpopular—in 1926 farmers refused to pick the crop—and production was not to pick up again until the build up to the Second World War at the end of the decade (Telford 1929; Bantje 1979: 38). But despite the drought and high flood of 1929–30, and more high flooding in 1932, rice sales remained large. This was one side of the response to the squeeze on reproduction. But because of the variability of the effects of flooding, just as some cropped bumper harvests, many others faced ruin, and 1930 saw a mass exodus from the district. As many as 5,000 people left to seek work in Dar es Salaam, Zanzibar, and Mafia, despite high unemployment in those areas (TNA 61/3/VI/D; Provincial Commissioner's Annual Report, Eastern Province, 1932).

The seriousness of the situation in the early 1930s can be seen in the fact that large-scale capitalist agricultural concerns in the district withdrew from production completely, an option not open to the people. The plantations, including four of sisal, lay abandoned (TNA 61/3/VI/D).

By 1933, with a good flood and a slightly higher cotton price, matters improved, and 1934 saw both a good rice harvest and the restarting of plantation agriculture. As the 1930s continued, producer prices gradually improved. However, a number of factors continued to limit the long-run growth potential of the district.

First, there was still a lack of investment in agriculture—in seeds, ploughs, or mechanization (TNA 61/3/IX/D; Bantje 1979). Second, ecological and environmental hazards were pervasive. Destruction caused by wild animals—elephants, hippo, pigs, monkeys, and birds—made all crop production vulnerable. This was in part a heritage of MajiMaji, which reversed the effects of the nineteenth-century ivory trade (Iliffe 1979: 201–2). However, it was exacerbated by the creation of the Selous game reserve in the south-west of the district in the 1940s, and also by an unbalanced approach by European hunters who killed crocodiles and lions, thereby disrupting the ecological chain, allowing smaller animals, such as pigs and monkeys, to proliferate.[3] Through the 1920s and right up to 1931 there are continual reports of damage (TNA 1733/1, 5; TNA 1733/17/1/10; TNA 1733/18: 105; TNA 61/3/VI/D). A systematic game control policy was only put into action in the early 1930s (RH, 1937), in which over 2,400 hippo were killed, and elephants were driven out of the Magongo Hills. This fell into abeyance in 1935 however (ibid.), and the problem returned. In 1986 there were still elephants in the hills. In addition to game, local locust plagues, floods, and famines recurred through the 1930s (Bantje 1980: 3–4).

A third impediment to economic expansion was the struggle over prices and debt with traders. Under the Germans, the trading system in Rufiji was the result of conditions that had favoured the Asian and Omani merchants, giving them a monopoly over both export and import trade, working under contract with the DOAG (Bantje 1979: 11). An estimate of profit rates on exporting produce to Dar es Salaam in 1920 was between 40 and 90 per cent, while the rate on imports was 30 per cent or higher (TNA 1733/1). With rates such as these, and with individual merchants making profits equal to over one-quarter of the annual district poll tax revenue, it was extremely hard for any producer to obtain a good return to labour, relative to world prices.

The British response was twofold: firstly, to encourage competition, and, secondly, to regulate usury and crop-purchasing practices. However, the two systems in operation—auction and bilateral agreement between farmer and buyer—still favoured the traders, who formed cartels (TNA 1733/18: 105). Smuggling of rice frequently occurred as a response (TNA 61/3/IX/D; Bantje 1980: 5). There was constant struggle between farmers and traders. The appearance of the larger trading companies on the scene did little to guarantee reasonable market prices for export crops such as cotton. Eventually, in 1943, marketing became completely centralized (TNA 1733/18: 105; Bantje 1979: 12). Further, over the course of the 1930s and 1940s, there was both horizontal concentration in trading, and vertical integration of marketing into processing and shipping in cotton, tobacco, and sugar (TNA 61/3/XIII/D; TNA 1733/18: 105).

Regulation may have curbed the worst excesses of mercantile exploitation. But the high rates of profit noted were possibly only because commodities had become so deeply rooted in the cycle of reproduction by the 1920s, both as crops sold, and as clothing and other items bought. Traders took full advantage of this fact and maximized their profits by exploiting seasonal price changes. They sent hawkers round the villages to persuade producers to sell both cotton and food at low, post-harvest prices. Later in the year, food shortages would drive people back to the shops, and food prices up. Some were driven into debt, and sold their crops forward. The extension of credit was in fact banned in 1919, and some control over food marketing was exer-

[3] Interview with Fr. R. Lamburn, Kindwitwi, Aug. 1986.

cised as part of famine-relief measures for the district. Nevertheless, debt continued to be a problem into the 1930s (TNA 61/3/VI/D; TNA 1733/1; TNA 1733/17/1/10).

A fourth constraint was transport. Transport infrastructure, both within the district, and linking the district with the Dar es Salaam market, remained a major problem throughout the pre-Second World War period. While the early axis of travel was from west to east along the river, by canoe (Bantje 1979: 11), the transfer of the administrative centre of the district to Utete in 1913 made road transport more important, and by 1921 there was a motor road from Dar es Salaam (TNA 1733/5; RH, i 1937). Nevertheless, throughout the 1920s road access was very poor, and crops were still transported by canoe (TNA 61/3/VI/D; TNA 1733/18: 105). The problem with large-scale river transport was the gradual silting of the delta. By 1931 the fortnightly steam tug service had ceased, and communication was henceforth to be by road, plagued by problems in the rainy season.

The district report for 1934 notes the paradox of exhortations to peasants to increase output while the means of transporting produce were totally inadequate. Accumulation through trade or agriculture was thereby hampered:

> The better class of Trader or Agriculturalist . . . hold back, or commence operations in less favoured but less cinderella-like areas. There are not 25 miles of properly drained road in the Rufiji, and not one permanent bridge to mark European occupation. Dar es Salaam—a mere 107 miles away—cannot be reached for nearly 6 months in the year except by air, and possibly 3 times during the period by coasting vessel from Salale. (TNA 61/3/IX/D)

Matters did not improve much until after the Second World War.

Finally, the development of large-scale capitalist agriculture in Rufiji—whether settler or Tanzanian—was additionally blocked by a lack of labour. Time and again the shortage of labourers from Rufiji for the few plantations is emphasized in the reports. After early futile attempts to aid plantation owners in the search for local labour, the district administration simply warned estate owners to recruit outside the district (TNA 1733/5; TNA 1733/17/1/10). The lack of labour supply was not uniform or total. In the case of one estate the problem was unpopular management, and sometimes people would work in the slacker seasons (TNA 61/3/XI/D). None the less, it was clear that it was through crop commodity production and migrant urban labour rather than agricultural wage or piece labour that the Rufiji peasantry were brought into the colonial economy.

Peasant–peasant wage labour relations were new to the district, and until today are sometimes perceived as a variant of mutual assistance (Telford 1929: 37). Plantation labour was of course strongly associated with the MajiMaji cotton scheme. But another reason for resistance was that, while both commodity production and wage labour in peasant agriculture are rested on cheap labour (Mamdani 1987: 193), in Rufiji returns to plantation labour were generally a lot lower than returns to labour in peasant production[4], and migration to Dar es Salaam.[5]

The Advent of Islam

In tandem with the growth in intensity of contact with the world economy and European imperialism, the people of Rufiji also converted to a major world religion—Islam—beginning in the mid-nineteenth century. By 1919 the whole district was Muslim (Trimingham 1964), and it remains the most uniformly Islamic part of rural Tanzania today.[6]

A key to understanding the spread of Islam, especially in the valley and delta, was the identity of being 'swahili'. As has been noted (Arens 1975; Westerlund 1980: 41; Caplan 1982: 29; Pouwels 1987), there are problems in defining a single criterion for swahili culture or ethnicity; it is rather a complex of religion, language, reckoning of descent, dress, and associated social structure. There has been constant redefinition of parts of what 'swahili' means, often by migrants from the interior who wished to assimilate themselves into the urban, Zanzibar-centred society of the coast.[7] However, a distinction can be made (and evidently was make contemporaneously) between *waswahili* proper, and the *wamrima*, those who were by the late nineteenth century indigenous dwellers of the coastal strip, but who retained ethnic identity as Zigua, Zaramo, or Rufiji (Burton 1860: 37–8; Tanner 1962: 81; Oliver 1977: 87). This ethnic distinction coincided with a normative one (for the *waswahili*), between the *wastaraabu*—the cultured people—and the *washenzi*—the uncivilized pagans.

In Rufiji, this distinction came to be associated with a difference between valley (and delta) and hills.[8] At the same time, a constant cultural movement was present over the whole Mrima coast in the late nineteenth century for political reasons, and as part of this many coastal *wamrima* adopted the malleable swahili identity in addition to upcountry immigrants (Glassman 1986: 5). The wearing of the *baibui* (veil), the 'Shirazi' or Omani ancestor, and the use

[4] For instance, in 1931 the average cotton price received was 16 cts/kg. From average yield figures, the cash return on one acre would have been around 38*s*. (Telford 1929: 23; Bantje 1979: 38). The figure for rice that year is difficult to gauge because the price is not known, but rice yields in 1931 were high. The number of person-days work required to cultivate one acre of cotton or rice, according to a 1929 study, was 37–8, and even less for *mlao* cotton (Telford 1929: 28). By contrast, with an unskilled agricultural wage rate of 50–60 cts/day, working as a wage worker for the same number of days would have netted 18–22 shillings. For 1936 the gap was larger: while one acre of cotton would have yielded around 58*s*., and rice around 60*s*., the equivalent wage work would have brought in 12–22*s*.

[5] While the 1936 unskilled agricultural wage was 8–15*s*. a month, the wage in domestic service varied between 10 and 80*s*. a month during the 1930s, and the wage for casual port labour was 16–30*s*. a month (TNA 61/3/XI/D; Tanganyika *Blue Books*).

[6] The town of Mohoro is an important religious centre.

[7] Westerlund 1980: 41–2; Glassman 1986: 5 gives the example of Mtoro bin Mwinyi Bakari (see Allen 1981) as an adopter of swahili identity. The example shows the role of the 'Shirazi' component in descent and swahili status.

[8] And a political one in Mafia, see Burton (1860), Caplan (1975), Swantz (1985: 23–4).

of Kiswahili were all possible signs of acquired status which spread contiguously with Islam, and particularly in the delta and lower river valley areas (Schacht 1965: 114; Swantz 1985: 23–4).

The attraction of Islam was therefore part of the attraction of being 'swahili'. However, it must be remembered that the Islam of Rufiji was deeply syncretic. It was also heterodox, with strong Sufic tendencies. In the first ten to fifteen years of British rule in Rufiji, this Islam provided an alternative and apparently hostile structure of political allegiance based around the Sufi *tariqa*: 'each area possesses several *waalim*, each with adherents and a banner, and each owing allegiance to a sheikh' (TNA 61/3/IX/D).[9]

The complex tension between the social conservatism and political radicalism of Islam continued to arise in a series of contradictory expressions in the post-war period. Muslims were prominent in the organization of the nationalist Tanganyika African National Union (TANU) movement (Iliffe 1979: 550–2). Yet there was an ambivalence in Islam about women's role in public politics, in this case simultaneously crucial but potentially dangerous. This can be seen in the case of Bibi Titi Mohammed, a Rufiji woman who effectively established TANU's mass membership in Dar es Salaam through the informal women's organization of the Muslim community, to the extent that in its first months the majority of the TANU members were women (Geiger: 1987). Despite her importance to TANU, and her eventual position as post-Independence head of the party's women's organization, there was often resistance to her public appearances (Iliffe 1979: 532; Geiger 1987). Such conflicts were played out on a wider basis as the new opportunities for expression for women in the Independence movement clashed with men's desire to maintain control over women.

With the dominance of Christian influence on the post-Independence government, especially through the Tanzanian Council of Churches and Nyerere himself, Islamic social concerns retained a form of political opposition, such as in the case of debate over the 1971 Marriage Act (Westerlund 1980: 161–71). This remains the case today, with social conservatism, and religious and political frustrations intermingling in a complex reaction, as for example in riots in Zanzibar in 1988.[10] At the same time, the heterodoxy and relative social radicalism of the *tariqa* possibly remains a key factor in limiting the influence of so-called 'fundamentalism'.

Migration to Dar Es Salaam

The quantitative data on patterns of migration from Rufiji to Dar es Salaam was presented in Chapter 1. It shows evidence of a small trickle of migrants to the city states from the nineteenth century, to Zanzibar early in the twentieth

[9] See also Eastern Province, Provincial Commissioner's Annual Report on Native Administration 1934 and RH, 'Notes on *dhikri*'.

[10] 'Poussée de fièvre à Zanzibar', *Le Monde*, 27/7/88; 'Rights riot', *Independent*, 17/5/88; 'Police killing', *Guardian*, 14/5/88; 'Muslim clash', *Times*, 14/5/88.

century, but increasingly to the growing city of Dar es Salaam. This flow greatly increased after the Second World War, in the period from the 1940s to the 1960s. Thus, in the pre-war and early post-war years, Dar es Salaam was a 'mainly uneducated, Muslim and coastal town' (Leslie 1963: 28). This overwhelmingly coastal nature of earlier migration gave parts of the city a distinctive cultural stamp, and made leaving home for urban life a less traumatic experience than might be thought. The people of Rufiji, coming along the Southern Route, maintained *utani*[11] relationships with the Wazaramo, out of whose hamlets and villages Dar es Salaam evolved. It was not an easy journey: before motor transport started in the 1940s, Rufiji migrants faced a two-to-three day march on foot. However, on reaching the city, they found the same religion, culture, and diet, even sharing political representation through the same *mashehe* with the Wazaramo (ibid. 20–1). Further, they came in sufficient numbers to establish supportive networks of relatives and friends: 'The Rufiji . . . are so numerous that nobody could lack for a relative to bury him; it might be equally argued that they are so numerous that nobody need feel alone' (ibid. 28).

Rufiji was not involved in labour migration to the north-eastern sisal estates, but many of the conditions and changes of the system applied similarly to the much more specialized labour migration from Rufiji to Dar es Salaam.[12] The district was a 'hybrid' area,[13] where people combined food production, export commodity production, and labour migration. Apart from geographical proximity, the main factor helping to channel Rufiji migrants towards DSM, as opposed to other destinations, was a heritage of political resistance to rural proletarianization. Combined with the existence of an alternative source of income in smallholding, this meant that peasants refused to work on plantations, both locally and elsewhere.[14] One colonial officer reported in 1924: 'I have no hesitation in affirming that the Rufiji native would rather do anything than work on an estate' (TNA 1733/17/1/10). Periodically, as world commodity prices slumped, not only labour supply, but also the labour demand from estates atrophied, as in the early 1930s (TNA 61/3/VI/D), and more or less permanently after the 1940s, as the unfeasibility of plantation production became evident.

The heyday of Rufiji migration was in the immediate post-war period. Migrants worked largely in the three main sectors of employment—transport, especially the port, construction, and domestic service. Just as in the rural sectors, urban employment relied almost exclusively on 'semi-proletarian' labour with high turnover in a system of circular migration, right

[11] *Utani* or 'joking' relations between ethnic groups facilitated mutual support for members of groups travelling through another group's, territory.

[12] For analyses of the migrant labour system in Tanzania see Beck (1980), Rodney (1981), Tambila (1981), Shivji (1986).

[13] For versions of the divisional structure of colonial Tanzania see Rodney (1981: 8) and Iliffe (1979: 274).

[14] TNA 1733/5; TNA 1733/18: 105; Provincial Commissioner's Report, Eastern Province 1931; TNA 61/3/IX/D; TNA 61/XI/D; TNA 61/504/1/II.

up until the 1950s (Shivji 1986: 107, 129). Already by the end of the war, however, similar concerns to those in the sisal industry—about low productivity and poor skilling levels—had come to dominate official views on urban labour. Three major reports in the 1950s identified the instability of the urban workforce rather than levels of employment, as the primary problem (Orde-Browne 1946; Bienefeld and Sabot 1972: 179–80). In both urban industries and in sisal, the proposed answer was the stabilization and regularization of labour (Rodney 1983: 27–8). This marked the beginning of the creation of a skilled, regular urban labour force, increasingly stratified over the years. As industrial and service employment diversified greatly, and the possibility of specialization increased with it, various contributing factors created a situation where Rufiji and coastal migrants tended to be concentrated in low-paid, unskilled, and often casual work, and in the 'informal' sector of the urban economy.

One of these was decasualization of labour arrangements in a range of industries, but especially of port labour, from the 1950s onwards.[15] The effect of decasualization on the structure of migration was substantial. A dichotomy arose between increasing real returns to a regular, especially skilled job, and decreasing returns to casual work, or work in an 'unskilled' job such as domestic service. In (decasualized) port labour and government employment, wages exceeded the rate of post-war inflation in the prices of sugar and kerosene, but relative wages in domestic service stagnated. A month's wage in 1957 could buy a domestic servant about the same amount of sugar as it could in 1927.

The contrast was even more striking for food prices. For rice, the picture is similar to that for sugar and kerosene—divergence between stagnant wages in domestic service and relative gains in the types of labour that were to be decasualized. The situation with maize is more dramatic, and maize generally eclipsed rice in importance as a staple urban food over the period. In the face of a wartime food crisis and accelerating post-war maize prices (Bryceson 1987: 169–70), wages in all sectors were squeezed. However, while the rises in nominal wages for government and port workers in the 1950s alleviated their position somewhat, the relative position of domestic servants became dire. At the low point of 1953, the domestic servant's wage could buy only 15 per cent of the maize it could have bought in the 1930s.

By the 1970s, a second generation of Rufiji migrants was coming to Dar es Salaam, but in increasingly different circumstances. First, the rate of urbanization increased, at least up until the mid-1970s (O'Connor 1988: 136–41). Second, employment in Dar es Salaam expanded rapidly, but not as rapidly as the labour force (Sabot 1979: Table 2.11; O'Connor 1988: 138). In 1967, 24 per cent of the Dar es Salaam urban population worked for wages; in 1978 it was only 16.9 per cent (Campbell 1985: 4). Third, from the late 1960s, a rapid upgrading of the middle-skill range of the urban labour force occurred, leaving those workers with little or no education (i.e. less than standard VII) at the bottom of the

[15] For a full account see Lockwood (1989*b*), which is based in turn on Mascarenhas (1970) and Iliffe (1970), as well as oral sources. For decasualization in the building trade see Shivji (1986). For struggles for better conditions and wages in domestic service see Shivji (1986: 107–9, 129) and Bujra (1987).

wage income distribution (World Bank, Basic Economic Report 1977, annexe III, app. B, tables 1–3).

Fourth, starting from an historical disadvantage in state education, Rufiji (and indeed most coastal) migrants had fallen behind other regional groups by the 1970s. The educational experience of potential migrants in post-war Rufiji may be contrasted with an area such as Kilimanjaro, where missionary activity meant relatively high missionary and state school attendance early in the century. By 1956 about 90 per cent of Chagga children were at school (Shann 1970; Iliffe 1979: 445). As late as 1967, primary school attendance in Coast Region was around 30–5 per cent for boys, and around 20 per cent for girls.[16] There was still some gap in the general population by 1978, at the inception of universal primary education. While around 44 per cent of those aged 10 and over in Kilimanjaro Region had some sort of state education—including 2.33 per cent in tertiary education—only 21 per cent of those in Coast Region had some state education, with 0.54 per cent in the tertiary sector (1978 Census, viii, Table 8.9).

While regional disparities in education were clear (and indeed were even worse for other regions), they were particularly marked in migrant populations, since it was the best educated from each area who tended to migrate. Through the 1960s, higher educational achievement was increasingly associated with a higher propensity to migrate to urban areas (Barnum and Sabot 1977: 115, table 1). In this situation, historical differences in education became sharper. Although Rufiji migrants were more educated than non-migrants, and second-generation Rufiji migrants were better educated than the first generation, they lagged behind other groups in the city. Thus, while 49 per cent of male migrants for Coast Region to Dar es Salaam in 1971 had no education, and only 2 per cent had secondary education, only 3 per cent from Arusha and Kilimanjaro had no education at all, and 34 per cent had studied up to secondary level (Bienefeld and Sabot 1972: Table 4.5).

These shifts had a considerable impact on the kinds of jobs that later Rufiji migrants obtained. The 'traditional' sectors of domestic service, construction labouring, and port work collapsed, from the late 1950s on. Because of the rapid growth of the city labour force relative to employment in the 1960s, and the problem of access to formal employment faced by relatively uneducated Rufiji migrants, there was an explosion in so-called 'informal' activity by migrants. In the 1971 NUMEIST survey, 58 per cent of Coast Region migrants were exclusively dependent on wages, by contrast with those from Arusha and Kilimanjaro, 74 per cent of whom were wage-earners.

Over the early 1970s, urban wage incomes declined in real terms by about 25 per cent, but incomes in the informal sector more than halved (Bevan *et al.* 1988: Table 3.13). While the initial growth in the informal sector was probably due to migrants attracted by the expansion of formal sector employment, by

[16] Egerö and Henin (1973: 126, table 7.11); see also M.-L. Swantz (1985: 34–6) for an account of the problems faced by girls trying to get access to education in Rufiji, even after universal primary education.

the late 1970s and early 1980s, lower incomes in self-employment diminished this flow.

By contrast, for those in government and other wage labour the 1960s and early 1970s were relatively good years.[17] The increase in real wages was due in part to settlement between the government and groups of workers, such as the dockers, as described above. However, with the growth of the informal sector, which depressed earnings in that sector, the surpassing of employment growth by growth in the labour force, and accelerating inflation, the 1970s and 1980s saw a precipitous fall in urban incomes. It is estimated that urban real incomes in 1984 had fallen to about 40 per cent of their 1969 value (Bevan *et al.* 1988: Table 3.15).

Challenges to the Polity

Some of the most important spatial and political reorganizations in Rufiji occurred with villagization in the 1960s and 1970s (see below), but attempts by administrations to replace lineage authority started much earlier. The British colonial administrative policy of Indirect Rule was based on the idea of rule through indigenous 'tribal' authority, which was taken to be centralized (and possibly hereditary). Often, as was the case in Rufiji, such political authority did not exist, and so the offices of 'Chief' and 'Sub-Chief' had to be created.

After the occupation of the key military and administrative centres of Rufiji in 1917, and formal trusteeship of Tanganyika from 1919, the British set about developing a system of political authorities (Jumbes) and jural control (Native Courts, introduced in 1924 and strengthened by ordinance in 1929).[18] Indirect Rule proper was started in 1927, but right up until the Second World War, British administration was plagued with passive resistance, tax evasion, and contempt of court—all practices based on a rejection of the legitimacy of British rule as externally imposed and as a centralized, hierarchical system (TNA 61/3/VI/D).

District and provincial administrators consistently associated the rejection of Indirect Rule officers with the political traditions of egalitarianism and decentralization.[19] At the same time, in the early years of Indirect Rule, the system whereby Jumbes were 'elected by the people' (TNA 1733/18/105) enabled lineage heads to manipulate the office through the election of unpopular, incompetent, and often young Jumbes whose authority could then be easily questioned.[20] The responses of administration to the Indirect Rule problem would have depended in part on the views held on the origin of the

[17] Two series of real wages can be constructed. One, from 1951 to 1963, is the government unskilled wage rate (Bryceson 1988) deflated by DSM RPI for wage-earners (*Statistical Abstract 1963*); the second, from 1966 to 1979 is the territorial minimum wage (Bryceson 1988) deflated by DSM low-income-earners RPI (United Republic of Tanzania, *Economic Survey* 1977/8 and 1978/9).

[18] RH, 'Notes on the History of Rufiji District'; Digest of Appeals from Local Courts (1953: 10).

[19] TNA 1733/17/10; TNA 61/3/VI/D; RH, 'Notes by R. V. Hartnoll'; Eastern Province, Provinical Commissioner's Report on Native Administration 1934.

[20] TNA 61/3/XIII/D; interview with Para Megge, 20.4.86, Mng'aru.

acephalous Rufiji polity. The policy of inaugurating 'tribal' leaders arose from the idea that Rufiji societies had only recently lost such offices, and only the recreation of structure was required to bring about control. Inevitably this led, aside from the general problems of resistance to Indirect Rule, to disputes over whether particular clans fell within the jurisdiction of this or that particular 'tribe'.[21] The alternative approach suggested, to base Indirect Rule on the system of land rights and recognized local lineage heads, was associated with the idea that Rufiji societies were originally decentralized (RH, 'Notes by R. V. Hartnoll'). In practice, and over time, a compromise evolved between social realities and British form. As early as 1925, before the start of Indirect Rule proper, councils of elders were formed beneath the Jumbes, in an attempt to obtain respect by devolving authority (TNA 1733/18/105). By the 1940s, the system of councils had emerged as the central plank of the 'tribal' authority policy, with executors (*mwenyemzi*) in Utete and Kikale, and at the lower level, a *mwakili* or *mtawala* for every locality or village (TNA 61/504/1/III).[22]

Changes in Spatial Organization

By the advent of Independence, two trends threatened to make settlement patterns increasingly untenable. The first is that larger floods were becoming more frequent. The second is that the axis of transport, trade, and communication with Dar es Salaam was shifting away from the river (which had become unnavigable by the 1930s) to the overland routes.

The problems of settlement patterns in Rufiji met dramatically with national political developments in 1968. In 1967, President Nyerere had called for the organization of *ujamaa* villages as part of a new approach to rural development policy in Tanzania. When the upstream villages were engulfed in a long, high flood in 1968, and 50,000 people lost their homes and crops, Nyerere made food aid conditional on the construction of new villages on the north bank, away from the floodplain (Turok 1975: 398). Setting up the first involuntary *ujamaa* villages in Tanzania, this directive anticipated the introduction of compulsory villagization on a national scale by five years.

To this extent, unlike the voluntarily formed *ujamaa* villages for the late 1960s, the Rufiji scheme represented an experiment in which the state tried to impose a suitable layout for *ujamaa* villages. Although people were consulted about the siting of the new villages, their layout was decided at the regional level. Each village was to hold about 250+ nuclear families, each family having a half-acre garden in the village, and a main *shamba* of three acres outside (Turok 1975: 400–6). Another flood disaster occurred in 1974, in which the downstream areas around what are now Mkongo and Ikwiriri were badly hit. Villagization in the areas took place under Operation Pwani (Bantje 1980: 9).

[21] Eastern Province, Provincial Commissioner's Annual Reports 1931, 1932.

[22] See also Iliffe (1979: 339–41).

Interpretations of villagization have varied since the inception of the policy. By 1974, when it had become clear that the *ujamaa* concept was not strong enough to promote mass voluntary village formation, the official justification became the concentration of population to allow more efficient and cheaper provision of services, such as water and health. Collective cultivation was originally to accompany collective settlement, but this was abandoned as unworkable. Nevertheless, it has been pointed out that villagization did allow increased control over cultivation by the state, and involved the reintroduction of minimum cropping requirements (e.g. Payer 1983: 794). Thus villagization can be interpreted as a strategy 'designed to increase government control over peasant farmers and to facilitate extraction of the surplus' in previously marginal areas, with the tacit support of the international 'development' agencies such as the World Bank (ibid. 796).

In Rufiji, one of the main effects of the villagization was to move people away from their fields, towards roads, and often to higher ground away from water sources. Bantje, writing at the end of the 1970s, feared that cultivation would cease altogether, and the villages become abandoned in mass migration to Dar es Salaam. Instead, possibly partly due to the ailing urban economy, it now seems that the strains placed on cultivation and water collection are part of the forces reversing villagization, as people in many places move back towards the river.

One good example is Chumbi, where I was conducting part of the migration survey in August 1986. The principal problem there was water shortage, and the consequent enormous amount of time required to gather water because of slowly filling wells. Women were using up to three hours a day just to collect water. As a result Chumbi was becoming progressively depopulated as people went back to their pre-1974 sites.

Economic Diversification

Because of the constantly changing conditions in Rufiji—the shift from river transport links to road, the uncertainty of flooding, fluctuating prices, long-term trends in migration opportunities—there has been considerable diversification in economic activities over the post-war period. The history of crop cultivation, extractive and craft activities reflects the constant search for better returns to labour, and for a reduction in labour intensity (both reflecting Yoshida's view that labour is a constraint on production in Rufiji).[23]

Neither rice nor cotton was a new crop on the coast when the colonial era began (Sheriff 1987: ch. 1), although cotton cultivation seems to have reached Rufiji only in 1900 (Bantje 1979: 5). In addition to rice, a large number of food crops were grown in both the pre-colonial and early colonial periods, especially in the downstream floodplain (TNA 1733/1; RH, 'Notes from Elton'). The

[23] Cited in Bantje (1979: 11).

cultivation of some of these crops, notably millet and sugar, declined in the face of colonial pressure to increase cotton and rice production. Millet has been replaced by maize in both the valley and hill-farming systems (TNA 61/3/VI/D; Bantje 1979: 5). In addition, under constant pressure and coercion from the authorities, cassava and bananas were grown as famine crops (Bantje 1979: 11 and 1980: 17–18).

Post-First World War cotton sales were moderate, but slumped after a crisis of confidence in the cotton price after 1926. Only after 1934, and the experience of migration and unemployment, did cotton output rise again, but after this date unprecedented sales were made, peaking in 1937 and 1940. After a preliminary peak in the late 1920s, and the disastrous flood of 1930, official rice sales reached ever higher peaks, culminating in the 1941 sales of almost 4,600 tons.

Throughout the pre-war period, rice remained a crop of central importance in the valley, for both food and sale purposes. It was regarded as the most valuable crop, with high returns to labour, and hence the 'main' crop (TNA 1924; RH 1942: vol. i; Bantje 1979: 4). Thus in the 1930s, rice sales were considered the normal or primary source of cash for the payment of tax. Over this period, the trend was towards the extension of cultivation over larger and larger areas (Table 4.1).

A similar trend is observable in the hill staple, maize. The acreage and harvest figures are, of course, very approximate, and in some cases on comparison

Table 4.1. *Acreage, harvest, and sales of rice and cotton, Rufiji District, 1925–1937*

Year	Acreage	Rice		Acreage	Cotton	
		Harvest (tons)	Sales (tons)		Harvest (tons)	Sales (tons)
1925	8,375	5,862	121	2,361	340	340
1926	n.a.	n.a.	n.a.	n.a.	n.a.	438
1927	9,500	7,000	632	100	12	12
1928	9,000	7,500	2,500	800	125	116
1929	5,000	3,000	687	3,000	182	170
1930	3,800	2,200	317	350	75	58
1931	10,000	5,500	3,000	5,000	75	48
1932	10,000	6,000	1,672	2,000	250	259
1933	10,000	n.a.	2,888	2,000	250	±400
1934	20,000	12,000	3,275	3,000	200	304
1935	9,000	6,000	1,400	3,000	600	578
1936	19,000	3,600	809	7,000	1,000	1,167
1937	19,000	3,600	1,899	8,000	2,500	2,135

Note: n.a. = not available.

Sources: Sales—Bantje (1979: 38); Harvests, Acreages—*Tanganika Blue Books*.

with the more accurate sales data, obviously wrong. None the less, acreage cultivated seems to have been growing.

Cotton was helped by high prices before the First World War and again in the 1960s, and was effectively enforced through various campaigns. What is striking over the long term is the complete stagnation of cotton production. After the most recent heydays of the early 1960s, cotton production has slumped in the late 1970s and early 1980s to the point where only one ginnery is operating, and where 123 bales were produced in 1982–3, compared with 985 in 1913 (Telford 1929: 12; Ofisi Mamlaka ya Pamba, Wizara ya Kilimo, Dar es Salaam).

By contrast, the 1960s and early 1970s were a boom period for cashew nut production. Cashews were introduced into the area in the 1950s, and production peaked in 1973–4, when the Coast Region provided 39,331 tonnes of

Table 4.2. *Purchases of cashews, 1961/2–1981/2, tonnes*

Year	*Tanzania*	*Coast Region*[a]	*Rufiji District*
1961/2	40,000		
1962/3	55,400		
1963/4	57,400		
1964/5	74,100		
1965/6	74,327		
1966/7	84,150		
1967/8	73,824		
1968/9	118,008		
1969/70	110,342		
1970/1	112,459		
1971/2	125,995		
1972/3	125,523		
1973/4	145,080	39,331	7,396
1974/5	118,947	30,574	5,013
1975/6	83,734	23,205	5,497
1976/7	97,645	19,176	5,068
1977/8	68,383	12,039	1,869
1978/9	57,068	16,853	1,678
1979/80	41,454	11,380	
1980/1	56,558	7,790	
1981/2	44,331	9,630	

[a] Excluding DSM.

Sources: Tanzania: 1961/2–1964/5—Bank of Tanzania, *Tanzania: Twenty Years of Independence: A Review of Political and Economic Performance*, DSM, n.d. table 28; 1964/5–1978/9—Frank Ellis, 'A preliminary analysis of the decline in Tanzanian cashew nut production', ERB Paper 79.1, UDSM (1980). app. table II; 1979/80–1981/2—*Statistical Abstract 1984*, DSM. Coast Region: 1973/4–1978/9—Ellis, table 1; 1979/80–1981/2—*Statistical Abstract 1984*, DSM. Rufiji District: Han Bantje, 'The Rufiji Agricultural System', BRALUP Research Paper 62 (1979): 6.

cashews, of which 7,396 came from Rufiji. By 1978–9, the figures were 16,853 and 1,678 respectively, and the decline went on into the 1980s (Table 4.2). This was due to a combination of a collapse in the real producer price, tree disease, and the dislocation of villagization in 1974.

In more recent years, the spread of agricultural and extractive activities in Rufiji seems to have expanded again, after the middle period when cotton, rice, and cashews were dominant. This is partly due to the movement of people into villages on higher land, further away from the *mlao* fields and the soils of the floodplain. As noted this has affected cotton particularly badly, and encouraged the growth of crops more suited to the terrace soils: cassava, legumes, sesame, etc.

Analysis of the mid-1970s implied that rises in returns to labour for men in fishing, craft production, extraction based on charcoal and forestry, and crops previously not marketed (especially pulses) meant a shift of their labour away from cashews, cotton, and rice (Havnevik 1983).

Some of these prices shifts were temporary: the relative price of cashews improved over the 1980s, while that of cassava went into a prolonged slough. However, charcoal prices have remained relatively high.[24] A new important sale crop emerging in the 1980s was citrus fruit, especially because it could be marketed informally. In 1986, some farmers in Mng'aru were selling oranges to the upstream villages, and providing limes for export the following day to Saudi Arabia.

Another factor has been shifts in the relative returns to different activities. Diversification and switching between activities has been a response to economic crisis. Overall, real rural incomes in Rufiji, as elsewhere in Tanzania, have fallen sharply since the beginning of the 1970s. Table 4.3 gives various indices of rural living standards from 1969 up to the early 1980s. The case of Rufiji is in fact worse than that suggested here, since the high 1976/7 figures are due to the temporary boom in the price of coffee, which is not grown in the district.

Havnevik (1983: 109–25) argued that falling terms of trade in Rufiji up to 1978, following the dislocation and productivity losses of villagization, coincided with an increase in marketed output in the district. Not only did this mean that there was a general intensification of the labour of both men and women, but it also meant that people were constantly changing activities in

[24] Sources for prices of crops are as follows (see also Lockwood (1989*b*: figs. 4.2 and 4.3).
Nominal prices
Paddy 1971/2–1984/5: Marketing Development Bureau (1986), *Producer Price Forecasts* (Vol. i, table 2), Dar es Salaam; 1985/6–1987/8: *Tanzania Economic Trends* 1, 1 (1988); Cotton (AR) 1971/2–1974/5: Bantje (1979: 38); 1975/6–1987/8: *Tanzania Economic Trends* 1, 1 (1988); Cashews 1971/2–1985/6: Marketing Development Bureau, *Producer Prices Bulletin* 5.8.85, Dar es Salaam; 1986/7–1987/8: *Tanzania Economic Trends* 1, 1 (1988); Cassava and Charcoal 1973/4–1978/9: Havnevik (1983: table 28); 1979/80–1985/6: Bryceson (1988) and own observations.
Cost-of-living deflators
1971/2–1975/6: Havnevik (1983: 113, 1970/1 prices).
1975/6–1987/8: *Tanzania Economic Trends* 1, 1 (1988, 1986/7 prices).

Table 4.3. *Indices of rural living standards, Tanzania, 1969–1982/3* (1969 = 100)

Year	I	II	III
1969	100.0	100.0	100.0
1970/1	—	—	—
1971/2	95.4	—	—
1972/3	92.6	—	—
1973/4	67.0	—	—
1974/5	61.7	—	—
1975/6	77.4	—	—
1976/7	100.9	135.6	135.6
1977/8	84.5	—	—
1978/9	66.6	—	—
1979/80	—	69.6	62.4
1980/1	—	—	—
1981/2	—	—	—
1982/3	—	67.9	55.1

Sources: I: rural income terms of trade—Havnevik (1983: table 25); II: rural incomes deflated by the official CPI—Bevan *et al.* (1988: 76, table 3); III: rural incomes deflated by a CPI adjusted to take account of parallel market prices—Bevan *et al.* (1988: 76, table 3).

the search for higher returns to labour as producer prices fell. The implication—that peasants could not 'withdraw' from the market and the state—was contrasted with Göran Hyden's 'uncaptured peasantry' argument (Hyden 1980).

5 Interpretations of Change

From the 1950s we have evidence of rising fertility in Rufiji, and more generally in the Coast. This was a moderate rise, from a low base, leaving total fertility rates in the 1980s still below those in other parts of Tanzania. Much of this rise is attributable to falls in primary and secondary sterility. Reductions in sterility were probably primarily brought about by developments in health care. An initial step was the campaign to eradicate gonorrhoea, which Brass (1987) argues was responsible for rising TFRs in Tanzania. Bantje (1988: 201) takes the view that holoendemic malaria, leading to a high level of stillbirths, has also been a major factor in low coastal fertility, so that the general improvement of health facilities after Independence, and again after villagization, would contribute to rising fertility.

However, the analysis of the proximate determinants of fertility in Chapter 2 suggested that other factors may have been involved. A rise in the marriage age for women, an increase in marital instability, and decreasing birth intervals are all implicated. In Chapter 3, evidence on the historical roots of marriage and abstinence was discussed, and major changes in Rufiji economy and society were traced in Chapter 4. In this chapter the various strands are drawn together in a set of interpretations of change in human, economic, and social reproduction.

Labour, Domestic Conflict, and Marital Instability

One of the arguments made in Chapter 3 was that a wide range of relations between husband and wife, encompassing household management, sexuality, labour, relationships with kin, and the state of the marriage itself, were embedded in each other. The nature of the economy in Rufiji, however, was transformed by the experience of colonialism. As described in Chapter 4, colonial policy and capital sought to restructure Rufiji into a mixed export crop-, food-, and labour-supplying area, but failed both to provide the investment and infrastructure to overcome barriers to a real growth in production and to seriously transform the relations of labour in the district.

Thus the history of agricultural production in Rufiji was one of constantly interrupted development. The value of crops rose and fell, and cultivation suffered from the vagaries of an uncertain ecology and an exploitative trading system. Periodically, marketing collapsed in the face of price falls or serious flooding and drought.

Several factors worked together to place particular strain on the household economy, and relations between men and women. One was the peculiarities of the cropping cycle, which led to conflicting demands on labour. Another was the general increase in labour intensity and demands which came with new crops and a greater planted area. Thirdly, because labour institutions were not transformed in the course of colonial and post-colonial economic change, family labour remained the basis of production. From an initially unequal gendered position, men increasingly attempted to control and appropriate the labour of women, especially their wives. At the same time, the meaning and management of divorce was changing under the influence of Islamic law. The resulting instability of marriage, evident in reports of conflict, separation, and divorce, became characteristic of the area.

Gender and labour relations

One of the major arguments of this chapter is that the gendered economy of Rufiji was eroded at specific points by the ingress of capital. Matters are complicated further by the partial absorption of a new cultural system—that of Islam—overlapping the period of economic colonization. A. P. Caplan has posited that the two were linked, that:

> [I]n those areas [along the East African coast] where a cash economy has become dominant, and particularly in areas where historical developments led to the formation of a class society, Islamic doctrine became a dominant ideology, and *mila* was accorded 'peripheral' status; . . . In other areas, . . . this happened to a much lesser extent. There were fewer economic changes, and . . . Islamic law was not rigidly applied. As a result, *mila* flourishes, not just as a 'peripheral' set of beliefs and practices, but as one given importance by the community of both men and women, even though it is the women who appropriate *mila*. (Caplan 1982: 40–1)

Here Islam is also especially associated with plantation agriculture, seclusion, and the withdrawal of women from production. Where women are working in agriculture, a dichotomy is drawn between the female 'subsistence' sector and the male 'cash' sector.

Ann Whitehead has argued for the significance of a different distinction, but one which may in fact overlap the cash/subsistence dichotomy proposed above. This is that between women working as independent producers and women working under male control as family labour (Whitehead 1990). As will be seen below, this distinction is related to Islamization, but here the extension of the cash economy was associated with the incorporation of women rather than their marginalization or exclusion from production.

The roots of the dual role for women lay in the duties and rights of husband and wife (and other relatives) in the gendered economy of the pre-colonial period. At the same time, there were routes by which agricultural surpluses circulated within the societies, some of which probably involved women working under the control of men, and young people under the control of older people. An early change was tax, which involved the extraction of surplus from the system, and hence any existing exploitative relations were bound to be intensified by it. The responsibility of payment fell nominally onto men (and this role was further legitimized by Islam), but this, along with the direct appropriation of male labour by the colonial state in porterage and road-building, became an element in new bargaining whereby women increasingly performed more labour for the family, and for men.

The forced cotton-growing scheme that precipitated the MajiMaji war placed heavy direct demands for labour on both men's and women's labour, and probably encouraged greater solidarity between men and women in the face of an obvious, external threat to livelihoods. Following the war and its aftermath, with the establishment of cotton as a smallholder cash crop, the locus of struggles over the control of labour shifted again. As plantation labour was never drawn to any significant degree from the district, the issue of subsumption of cultivation under commercial control never became an issue (as it had done during MajiMaji). It did mean, however, that the subsumption of women's labour on cotton crops marketed by their husbands was much easier (TNA 1733/18:105; Telford 1929: 26).

We saw in Chapter 4 that the period between the wars was one of a broad trend of increase in farmed area and sales of cotton and rice. Harvests and sales fluctuated greatly according to production conditions and prices. The consequences for domestic relations can be seen in the two dimensions of seasonal and long-term change. In the absence of factors such as ploughing or fertilizer-use giving a systematic shift in productivity, increases were made possible only by a greater intensity of labour. Because of the timing of planting and harvesting, rice and *mlao* cotton were often conflicting in their labour demands, partly explaining the occurrence of rice and cotton peak harvests in different years (Bantje 1979: 11). Rice was the most valuable food crop, as was recognized at the time (TNA 1733/1), and was for most of the time more valuable than cotton. Yields varied with flooding and rainfall, but the rice yield per acre was about two or three times that of cotton in weight, while their labour intensity was about the same (Telford 1929). Therefore, unless the relative producer price of rice was very low, as for example in 1940, rice production was to be preferred. During the 1930s as a whole, cotton was probably just better value than rice only when its price hit 20 cts/kg. and above, i.e. 1936–7.

As noted, variation in harvests of cotton and rice from year to year depended on flooding and rainfall, and the two crops tended to complement each other in any one year. Rice harvesting in May–June conflicted with cotton interplanting, and while an early flood favoured rice and not cotton, a late flood favoured cotton and not rice. Cotton was harvested in November, around the time of preparing fields for rice-planting.

All cotton harvested had to be sold or thrown away, and so was entirely a cash crop. Cotton planting depended upon the flood and the rice harvest, and, perhaps secondarily, on the cotton price. By contrast, it was rice sales that depended upon the cotton harvest, since rice could also be eaten as a staple or in celebrations. Rice planting and harvests were probably more or less independent of cotton prices or harvests. This was to have important consequences for gender relations in farming, for while cotton cultivation was fully supervised and partly done by men, rice came to be much more of a woman's crop. Control of women's labour, either directly on cotton if the rice had failed, or indirectly in the form of rice to be sold if the cotton had failed or was not planted, was therefore a key point of conflict.

Marital instability in an Islamic context

It is important to stress again the bargaining and potentially conflictual nature of gender relations here, and the ideological aspect of this is considered below. In this process, the outcome often reflected the relative strengths of the partners. For example, an older, divorced woman in an informal union would be in a better position than a young woman in her first marriage (Swantz 1985: 38). And conflict it clearly was, with the threat of domestic violence certainly present. In Tanner's study of gender relations in Tanga in the late 1950s, the single most frequent reason for women bringing a case to court was assault (Tanner 1962: table 1).

In these circumstances, many women sought to end their marriages, just as many men sought to use marriage and quick divorce as a means to control women's labour, without long-term loss of the resources they would have to give in marriage payments (TNA 1733/17/1/10; TNA 1733/18:105). The legal context of family issues, such as marriage, adultery, divorce, and inheritance progressively passed out of the lineage sphere towards that of Islam: from the rules of *mila* to the rules of *sheria*. This process was selective, according to the issue, but Islam is clearly important in explaining the establishment of a high divorce rate regime along the East African coast (Landberg 1986: 113).

Within the syncretic culture of the coast, Islamicization led to a dual system of ideologies and practices in law and religion. On the one hand was *mila*—the customary laws and relations, which stressed communal rights and relative gender equality—and on the other was *sheria* or Islamic law. *Sheria* involves individual property rights and is based on a moral system in which women are inferior to men (Trimingham 1964; Knappert 1970; Caplan 1982: 30, 38–40, and 1984: 24–5).

Religion in Rufiji is still clearly syncretic—pre-Islamic practices and beliefs persist, and few people follow all Quranic precepts. However, constant tension exists, and it was in the area of family law and relations that Islamic authorities in Tanzania were most concerned to impose their influence (Schacht 1965: 113); family law was the 'very kernel' of *sheria* (Westerlund 1980: 167). As a result, family law and relations became progressively individuated, and within this marriage became individuated, and its meaning changed. From being primarily an almost political institution with important implications and consequences for a number of people related to bride and groom, it acquired a new identity as a *contract* between two individuals. In this sense Islamic marriage is also different from Christian marriage, with the latter's status as religious sacrament (Caplan 1984: 32).

A good example of the ways in which social control over domestic relations was transformed by Islam is adultery. Not only in Rufiji, but also along the coast (Tanner 1962), adultery was seen as increasing in frequency during the colonial period. Sanctions against adultery developed from loosely organized killings into a lineage controlled matter; arbitration over a domestic conflict became an issue between two groups (RH, 'Native Customs'). As such, the lineage membership of all parties was stressed above their identity as domestic individuals. Over time, and with the spread of Islam, adultery developed further into an issue between individuals (husband and wife, or husband and wife's lover), before an impersonal court.[1] However, within the domestic group, since a wife cannot divorce a husband on grounds of adultery alone in *sheria*, a diminishing of the significance of lineage membership coincided with the strengthening of an *unequal* individual identity for men and women.[2]

It was on family matters that Islamic law was probably most widely accepted by the colonial courts as 'customary' law. In general, the administrators had a greater affinity for *sheria*, as a written corpus of law, than for *mila*, based on oral custom. Although the frequency of conflicts arising from this structure was well known to the administration, the District Commissioners and the Court of Appeal tended to take every opportunity to reinforce the position of *sheria*. The colonial legal system, in harmony with the philosophy of Indirect Rule, was based on the application of 'traditional' or 'customary' law, except where it clashed with 'British' principles of justice or fairness. Wherever the appellant and the respondent were identified as Muslims of the same school, the Islamic law of that school was considered appropriate, and the case was heard by the *liwali*, no matter how nominal the ascription of 'Muslim' was.

This shift had various implications for women. Examination of the appeals from local courts shows the difficulties faced by women in obtaining divorce under *sheria*.[3] It had to be induced rather than claimed directly. Nevertheless, it was possible: simply by leaving and obtaining a divorce by default, or by bargaining for a divorce by the practice of *khula*, which is described as 'a repurchase of herself by the wife for a consideration'.[4] One of the most frequent grounds for suing for divorce given by women was failure of maintenance (e.g. Tanner 1962: 71, 79), an expression in legal form of the dissatisfaction of women at being drawn too far into family labour at the expense of their own agricultural and financial independence, in a situation where their husbands were not contributing.

Rice and the diversification of the male economy

As described in Chapter 4, apart from a brief period in the 1960s, cotton cultivation in Rufiji failed to take off, and the 1970s and 1980s saw a considerable diversification of activities in pursuit of better returns. Almost all of these

[1] Ibid. It is also interesting to note that Kinjikitile (the main ideological figure in the MajiMaji uprising) is said to have denounced adultery on religious grounds in a series of edicts in the years leading up to 1906 (Gwassa 1972: 212).

[2] Islam also deleteriously affected women's participation in public politics, since Islamic offices were all held by men, and the religion prescribed segregation of women to 'non-public' (i.e. non-male) space (e.g. TNA 1733/18: 105). However, this does not mean that women lost all political influence or participation, and probably also increased the political significance of women's ritual.

[3] Tanganyika, *A Digest of Appeals from Local Courts*, i–iv (1930–57), Dar es Salaam.

[4] Ibid., iv. 4.

were activities done by, or controlled by, men. The diversification of male labour was not accompanied by a similar shift for women, except possibly into charcoal. Their labour still centres around cassava, maize, and above all rice. As a result, men grew less rice, and acreages have fallen. Today, this means that fields are cleared later in the year than they were previously, and the consequently longer 'slack' season is taken up with fishing, charcoal, trading, and other labour. The reasons for the differential response of men and women is complex. One key factor is villagization. Over the longer term, the differential impact of the new settlement pattern for men and women took a different form for the upstream and the downstream areas (Bantje 1979: 35). The upstream villages, having changed to the north bank, were cut off from the floodplain by the river. Old fields were now difficult to reach and exposed to wild animals, and rice cultivation ceased, leaving only *mlau* cotton. These villages essentially turned towards Dar es Salaam, as have some of the larger villages downstream on the north side of the river. Since rice is an important crop for women, this has placed them under a particular pressure. In response they have tried to find new niches: in production and trading of cooked foods; in craft production for sale; in brewing.

The downstream villages have retained access to the floodplain, but now at a greater distance (Bantje 1979; Swantz 1985: 43). This has led to a sharp bifurcation of men's and women's economies. While men have more or less abandoned cotton and their minor role in floodplain rice, and thrown themselves into a second agricultural system of cashews, cassava, and simsim, women have found themselves facing longer distances to get to the fields, and longer stays away from the villages, the markets, and the lines of communication. Underlying the effects of villagization are gender divisions of tasks which proscribe women from those activities with higher returns: such as fishing, logging, bicycle repair, tailoring, etc. (Havnevik 1983: 55–7). Another factor is that expected contributions to the family pool are often gender-specific—men providing money and women labour.

However, the right of women to earn and keep an independent income has not disappeared, and the basis for this independence has largely continued to be rice for a number of reasons. First, although there are fluctuations, the relative price of rice has held up over the last fifteen years. This is even on official prices, whereas much of women's marketing of rice is on the parallel market where rice prices are substantially higher. Thus, although women often retained only part of the rice crop for sale on their own accounts, this portion still had a high value.

Underlying these economic facts was the more basic ideological status of rice, even today, as a 'women's crop' (Swantz 1985: 39). This is partly because of the nature of the process of growing rice in Rufiji, and the specialization involved. Rice, whether rain-fed or floodplain, requires the cultivator to live in the fields, away from the centres of marketing, transport, and communications for several months of the year. Male extractive activities, such as fishing, and later logging and charcoal, as well as migration, kept men away from the rice fields. They were not heavily involved in the cultivation, and could not supervise women so closely. As a result male claims to rights over the proceeds from rice could not be legitimized so easily, although this did not stop such proceeds becoming an issue of conflict (ibid.: 39–40). The other major difference between rice and the alternative valuable crop—cotton—is that rice could be marketed informally and locally, giving more scope to women for the independent realization of their product.

Growing rice is very important for women. Many who live in Kibiti, which has little suitable rice land near by, grow rice in the valley beyond Mng'aru. This involves regular and frequent journeys by foot of ten kilometres, transporting food, tools, cooking pots, and so on. Despite these difficulties, women continue to devote large amounts of labour time to this cultivation.

Abstinence and Domestic Conflict

In Chapter 3, two interpretations of the course of abstinence behaviour in Rufiji were proposed. One was that abstinence had previously been maintained by a cosmological sanction, threatening danger if sex and breastfeeding were linked, but that such a 'taboo' has been eroded over the twentieth century. The second was that there was no evidence that such a link had existed in the past, but rather that there was an avoidance of *pregnancy* and breastfeeding before sufficient development of the index child and weaning.

As noted in Chapter 3, one problem with the first interpretation is the absence of teaching of any kind of 'taboo' linking sex and breastfeeding in any accounts of rite. A further problem lies in explaining why such a shift should occur, given the resilience of elements of cosmology in Rufiji and elsewhere along the coast.

This can be seen in the experience of MajiMaji. The ideology of MajiMaji drew heavily on the early twentieth-century syncretic cosmology of south-eastern Tanzania, incorporating elements of Islam into a hierarchy of deities and humans, and an ordering of men and women in the natural world. It would seem at first sight likely that this cosmology received a severe blow with the crushing of the rebellion, and the evident failure of the *maji* to protect men against bullets. And yet the symbols and the components of witchcraft belief remain, including the potency of *maji*, as does the belief itself. Furthermore, whereas we might argue that the collapse of the old belief system accounted for the rapid spread of Islam between 1907 and 1920, it is important to remember that MajiMaji was not pre-Islamic. If MajiMaji was a blow to belief, why not to Islam as well, since there were Islamic elements in it (Iliffe 1967: 499; Gwassa 1972: 212)?

Indeed, if cosmologies have changed, and if elements of rite have been abandoned, the most likely immediate agent of change is Islam. On Mafia, those who did not put their children through *unyago* were the Islamic élite, the *Masheikh* (Caplan 1976: 29). Islam does provide a clear teaching on post-partum sexual abstinence, with a forty-day period. This influence is widely referred to in the area (Cross-Upcott 1956: 268–9; Swantz 1970: 100, 185, 191, 197, 284, 326; Caplan 1976).[5]

Understanding change in birth spacing on the second interpretation takes us in a somewhat different direction, one that emphasizes again conjugal conflict and the embeddedness of sexual and economic relations. Conflicts over rights to labour and product, through the periodic intensification of commodity production, became expressed not only directly in a breakdown of the overall marital relation—separation and divorce—but also in the sphere of sex and breastfeeding.

Breastfeeding has a contraceptive effect, but one which is entirely dependent on the frequency and intensity of suckling. This tends to fall off as the infant grows older. The earlier the resumption of intercourse, and the more frequent it is, the earlier the next conception is likely to be. If there is no 'taboo' linking sex with breastfeeding, these factors will be bound up with the general relations between husband and wife.

In the pre-war period, economic conflict between husband and wife was over labour on cotton. In the post-war period, as men turned away from the floodplain towards the city and the hills for their livelihoods, the struggle became increasingly to do with control over rice itself. A movement away from cooperation towards conflict was also accentuated by Islam, which was providing two new messages. One was the importance of the individual, rather than the lineage. The other was the separateness and therefore the strength, of gender identities. As Caplan notes for Mafia, the increasing segregation of women at funerals, marriages, religious festivals, and even in village events, while it clearly effectively excludes women from public space and overt power, 'may actually give women "a space of their own" in which to develop their own rituals' through which to 'make their presence felt' (Caplan 1982: 34).

Thus Islam may not only have individuated, but also have strengthened collective gender identity by giving a more gender-specific focus to ritual and ceremony. These events were and are also extra-household, and to an extent sometimes external to lineage. In Uzaramo, we see a shift from clan or lineage rites to an emphasis on gender (e.g. Swantz 1970: 308, 331).

As individual interest became more accentuated, so did the transactional element in sexual relations, discussed in Chapter 3.[6] Women were not only increasingly in more individuated positions, but also under greater economic pressure. Caroline Bledsoe has considered such a situation in contemporary Sierra Leone, where it is avoiding sex, rather than pregnancy, that is linked to lactation:

[5] Islam has also had an impact on male circumcision, which is now carried out earlier.

[6] A transactional element of sex is argued by Caldwell *et al.* (1989) and Standing and Kisekka (1989: 5, 54) to be widespread in Africa.

Generally . . . people relate early weaning and resumption of sexual relations less to women's desire for a new pregnancy than to increasing economic and social pressures. Women face growing demands for cash . . . A woman can press her demands with far greater leverage if she is not sexually and domestically remote. (Bledsoe 1987: 109)

Such dynamics can be seen in the seasonal pattern of births (and conceptions) in the Rufiji village of Ikwiriri. Examining records from a Swedish mission hospital between 1972 and 1984, Bantje (1988) finds a peak of conceptions in the period November to January at the beginning of the rainy season. This is the period when the rice from the July harvest begins to run out, and if the short rains fail, there can be food shortages:

During that time, women become more dependent on cash earning males and there is no doubt an association between financial assistance and sexual favours. Midwives in Ikwiriri made the observation that sexual intercourse at a late stage of pregnancy is often responsible for stillbirths. When told to abstain from sexual favours at that stage, women reply 'What shall I eat then?' This suggests that the increased dependence of women on men during the period of habitual food shortage (November–February) may underlie a higher incidence of conceptions at that time. (Bantje 1988: 199)

A Transformation of the Marriage System?

In Chapter 3 I argued that marriages partly played the role of forging alliances between the scattered hamlets which made up Rufiji society before the transformations of colonialization and villagization. Marriages thus involved a number of different relationships: between the potential bride and groom; between the groom and the bride's parents and family; between the bride and her parents; and between the two families.

Any factors which acted to disrupt these sets of relationships would tend to delay marriages and reduce the incidence of first marriage. Any factor which acted to bypass these relationships, or render them redundant, would transform the marriage system itself, and could act to lower or raise the average female age at first marriage.

Marriage, space, and politics revisited

Probably the most radical disjuncture of the system occurred with villagization. However, the early part of the century saw large-scale disruption caused by forced-labour schemes, war, famine, and epidemics, occurring sporadically but frequently between the 1890s and 1930.

Material and political disruption, which delayed marriage (Cross-Upcott 1956: 208–9; Bantje 1980: 11), affected the cohorts moving through these years. With constant movement disrupting the management of alliances, and shortages preventing the conducting of ceremonies and the accumulation of marriage payments, the first years of the century may well have seen a rise in marriage ages for both men and women.

The link between marriage, space, and politics faced its largest upheaval during villagization. Villagization emerges as a particularly important turning point because of the timing of the rise in marriage ages noted in Chapter 2, since it occurs between 1967 and 1978. Not only was this exactly the period of villagization in Rufiji, but it precedes the beginnings of education for girls through universal primary education.[7]

Villagization gathered together the small, lineage hamlet groups, and saw the formation of centralized villages under the political jurisdiction of government and CCM party officials. At the same time, villagization, especially in the utilization of the *ujamaa* concept, led to a partial redefinition of domestic relations. The ideology of villagization, as Goulbourne has pointed out, was encapsulated in the idea of the *unity* of the family: 'For Nyerere, the family in African traditional society was a harmonious unit within which there was no fundamental rift reflecting particularistic interests: the interest of the individual was also the interest of the whole' (Goulbourne 1978: 383).

In particular, *ujamaa* was in theory based on the assumptions of mutual respect, obligation to work, and commonly held and shared property (Nyerere 1968: 107–9). What is interesting is that the *ujamaa* ideology was practically applied in a villagization programme which effectively favoured the organizational form of nuclear families under male control, at the expense of both lineage authority and women's independent productive base. Thus villagization had a centrifugal effect on lineage power, diverging it both upwards and downwards, to village government on the one hand, and to families on the other. Villagization created fewer, larger communities. Marriage alliances were created between fewer, more concentrated locations, and were also more likely to be made within a village.

In Cross-Upcott's study of a Kingindo settlement in the 1950s, one-third of spouses came from within the settlement, one third from within twenty-five miles, and one-third from more than twenty-five miles away. He argues that this is probably unusually concentrated for Ungindo (Cross-Upcott 1956: 118–9).

As part of a birth and marriage history survey in the created village of Ikwiriri, married women were asked about where they had lived before marriage. Women had married in from a wide range of locations, but over 50 per cent came from the two locations of Ikwiriri–Ndundu corridor and from Dar es Salaam.

The idea of lineage is still important in Rufiji. But, as lineage alliances and control on the one hand, and the geographical dispersion of friendly kin on the other became less important, the system started to lose respectively its means and its ends. There is less pressure on young men and adolescent girls to marry. At the same time, resistance to such control has grown. Certainly since the advent of education for girls, from the early 1980s onwards,

[7] This in any case took some time to implement in Rufiji, because of parental resistance (Swantz 1985).

schooling has become a factor. However, the nature of generational relationships has also changed.

Generational relations

The history of generational relationships is also bound up in the history of political transformations. We saw in Chapter 4 that Indirect Rule ended in a stalemate between the imposition of 'tribal chiefs' and the persistence of lower levels of lineage-based authority.

The general failure of the implementation of Indirect Rule to stateless societies led the colonial authorities to the belief that in the past, civil and domestic power had coincided. Concerned with political stability, the administration brought family and Indirect Rule policy together in an attempt to enhance male parental authority as the basis for civil and government authority (TNA 1733/17/10).

This can be seen in the way in which the colonial state moved against various challenges to the rule of the old over the young through the institution of lineage. One such challenge came from a heterodox, Sufic Islam (see Chapter 4). At the same time, the challenge to parental and gerontocratic authority ultimately came from the 'conceited youth'. The period between the wars was one of change in the structures and opportunities facing young men. As juniors, their relationships to elders of lineage and family were affected by continuing commoditization, and especially by the growth of Dar es Salaam as a migration destination. Juniors successfully used the colonial jural system to challenge parental rights to use corporal punishment, and also used their organizations—the *ngoma*, or dance societies—in political ways, as in Ndundu in the 1930s (TNA 1733/17/10; RH, 'Dance societies in Ndundu').

Generational relations were also strongly affected by changes in the form of marriage payments and the ability to pay them independently of kin. Cross-Upcott (1956: 206) points out that even by the 1950s, substituting cash payment for the system whereby suitors would go and work on their prospective in-law's farms was a longstanding practice. Marriage payments were constantly rising, and the bridegroom would usually need the close involvement of kin, but 'Nowadays to an increasing extent, thanks to migrant-labour, the suitor seeks his own bridewealth' (ibid. 218).

Very early marriage for girls in Rufiji and surrounding areas was part of a system in which controlling marriage was key, and in which 'groups try to secure marriage partners in advance and to indoctrinate them thoroughly' (Cross-Upcott 1956: 257). This system was changed abruptly with villagization, but the introduction of universal primary education for girls as well as boys in 1977 still met with great resistance as parents constantly tried to remove daughters from school (Swantz 1985: ch. 1). Nevertheless, this further instance of the reshaping of political and domestic relations in Rufiji has created further space for teenage girls to assert their own wishes on when they will marry.

Table 5.1. *Polygyny in Coast region/Eastern province, 1957–1978*

Year	Percent of married men by number of wives			Ratio of currently married women to men
	1	2	3+	
1957	76.3	19.9	3.8	—
1967	—	—	—	1.2
1973	77.2	19.6	3.2	—
1978	—	—	—	1.18

Sources: Tanganyika, *African Census Report 1957* (1963), Dar es Salaam, 78; United Republic of Tanzania, Bureau of Statistics, *1967 Population Census* (1971), vol. 3: 57; United Republic of Tanzania, Bureau of Statistics, *NDS*, i: 159; United Republic of Tanzania, Bureau of Statistics, *1978 Population Census* (1982), vol. 7: 17.

Polygyny

A final point needs to be made with regard to polygyny. Polygyny is commonly associated with lower fertility and sterility.[8] It is also obviously associated with a male–female age difference at marriage and generally with a young age at marriage for women. If levels of polygyny had fallen since the 1950s, this might in part explain a rise in female age at first marriage, and an increase in fertility. However, available evidence from census data suggests that there has been no change in a level of polygynous marriage that is on the low side for Africa.

In 1922 the British introduced a tax on 'plural wives', i.e. on polygyny (TNA 1733/5; Shivji 1986: 12). This remained in force until the early 1950s (Cross-Upcott 1956: 224). Cross-Upcott claims to have found a rapid *increase* in the proportion of polygynous married men in Ungindo, from some 15 per cent of taxpayers in the early 1940s to 38 per cent in 1952.

However, regional data from 1957 to 1978 show little evidence for either a clear rise or fall in rates of polygynous marriage (Table 5.1).

[8] e.g. de Jonge and Sterkenburg (in Egerö and Henin 1973: 251–2). However, the level of association is often small (Pebley and Mbugua 1989).

PART II

Introduction to Part II

In the second part of this book I examine the influence of household demography on the work of men and women in a Rufiji village—Mng'aru. Why should demography matter for work and accumulation patterns? In most analyses of demographic and economic interaction, it is assumed that economic factors, such as prices and wages acting on the opportunity cost of time, determine demographic decisions. However, one premiss underlying this book is that fertility behaviour in Tanzania cannot be seen in terms of such economically determined decision-making, and that for the purposes of examining current labour allocation, it can be regarded as exogenous. Other demographic events, such as marriage, household extension and fission, and mortality, are more likely to be determined by economic factors. The result is that while in the long run households can adapt demographically in certain ways to changing economic circumstances, in the short run they are largely constrained by their current demographic composition.

This approach appears at first sight to resemble a model of the rural economy put forward by Chayanov. Since there are a number of controversies attached to the use of Chayanov's ideas in an African context, and since my approach is in fact distinct, and more general than Chayanov's, it is worth describing that model and the associated controversies in some detail.

Chayanov and Lenin

The work of A. V. Chayanov was extensive, combining a detailed analysis of the organization of the peasant farm in Russia with an account of the relationship of the farm sector to the national economy (Chayanov 1966). Comprehensive accounts and critiques are readily available elsewhere (e.g. Hunt 1979; Harrison 1982; Shanin 1987; Rahman 1988). Here I am concerned with the central and most characteristically Chayanovian element of his work—namely the influence of household composition on the scale and intensity of economic activity.[1] The importance of household composition flows immediately from Chayanov's central observation about peasant economy—the absence of wage labour. Since, without hired labour, 'the labour force pool, its composition and degree of labour activity are entirely determined by family composition and size, we must accept family make-up as one of the chief factors in peasant farm organisation' (Chayanov 1966: 53).

[1] As Hunt (1979: 247) points out, the arguments about differentiation and mobility follow on from these considerations about household resource allocation.

As the household cannot hire wage labour, and since, Chayanov argues, work has disutility attached to it, resource allocation, and in particular, the minimum amount of work required, is set by the needs of the absolute number of people in the household. The amount of work any one (working) person does then depends on the ratio of consumers to workers in the household. If a household has a high dependency ratio, the workers in it will have to work harder, or longer hours, than those in a household with a lower dependency ratio (Chayanov 1966: 60, 76–8). However, absolutely larger households have an advantage, because the presence of many members allows specialization and greater efficiency—what Chayanov calls 'complex co-operation' (ibid. 60). The requirements of a larger family also involve the cultivation of more land, and Chayanov argues that where land is in flexible supply, through renting or 'communal repartitioning', there will be a positive relationship between sown area and household size (ibid. 61, 132).

Both family size and consumer/worker ratios change over the course of the life cycle, so that the life cycle then becomes a major determinant of differences in observed farm scale and income. While the household gradually but continuously grows in size, its consumer/worker ratio first rises and then falls (Chayanov 1966: 59):

> Thus, every family, depending on its age, is in its different phases of development a completely distinct labour machine as regards labour force, intensity of demand, consumer-worker ratio and the possibility of applying the principles of complex co-operation. (Chayanov 1966: 60)

Chayanov's work is usually contrasted with that of Lenin, who saw the Russian rural economy as undergoing a polarization into landowning and landless households, with the latter performing wage labour for the former. Hours of work were determined by wealth, not consumer/worker ratios. Economic mobility was not cyclical, related to household expansion and contraction, but rather was polarizing, based on the extraction of surplus value through wage labour (Lenin 1972). Underpinning their arguments were different approaches to basic institutions of the rural economy governing land and labour. Chayanov's analysis assumes that there is no wage-labour market, and that land is freely available. Lenin, on the other hand, argued that wage labour was widespread and that large numbers of rural households had no access to land.

Subsequent Developments

The fundamental issues from these two views have now been taken beyond debates about the Russian peasantry into general analyses of labour allocation and household mobility.

On the Chayanovian side, household composition and its effects on economic activity have been taken up more recently by those studying the value of children. Some of the earliest work on children's labour inputs was done by Ben White in Indonesia. In comparative work on Indonesia and Nepal, White and others redeployed the complex cooperation argument, pointing out that larger households had more 'surplus' time over household tasks, and that the role of children's labour in freeing adult's time and thereby increasing efficiency of the household was key (Nag *et al.* 1980).

Their argument was thus that the smallest households, with the fewest children, were the poorest because they had the least surplus labour. However, this interpretation was challenged by Terence Hull, who argued that larger families have more opportunities and therefore are economically busier, because they are richer, rather than the other way round. Their greater wealth means that they can invest in productive capital, giving them higher productivity and higher returns to labour, and therefore an incentive to work more (Hull 1980: 273).

Hull's argument is an instance of how Lenin's criticisms of Chayanov are still applied to explanations of economic mobility based on household demography. A good example of this approach applied to household labour allocation is Gillian Hart's work in Java (1980). She starts from the observation from other studies in Asia that the poorest groups tend to work the longest hours (Hart 1980: 191). Time spent in economic work, as opposed to housework, depends upon its productivity, and hence wealth and access to inputs, and upon the ability to hire labour (ibid. 193). Defining class by asset ownership, she then finds in her own data a basic pattern of inter-class differences in labour allocation, whereby people in the poorest households do more economic work and less housework, but their returns to labour are lower than those in the richer group. People in richer households do less economic work, but hire labour in to do it (ibid. 201–4). Most importantly, this relationship holds even when class differences in household composition are taken in account (ibid. 207).

What emerges quite clearly from these contrasting views on labour allocation in the peasant household is that much depends on the arrangements governing land and labour. As Chayanov himself notes, his model is premissed not only on the absence of hired labour, but also on flexible land supply:

> [W]here . . . the land regime makes land use somewhat immobile, we encounter the land area as a determinant, even in family farms. Disharmony between family labour force and area worked is regulated either by hiring a workforce and going to work on the side. . . . But in countries where the land regime makes the land area extremely mobile, the determining significance of 'available' area falls to zero. Communal repartitions, long-term and short-term rentings and . . . purchases and sales permit adequate adjustment of size of land for use to the farms requirements. (Chayanov 1966: 132)

By contrast, Gillian Hart's work was carried out in rural Java, where 'a large proportion of the population is either landless or near landless', and where there is consequently a large agricultural wage-labour market (Hart 1980: 191).

Chayanov's work might thus appear to be of limited relevance, applying to the special situation where operational landholdings respond to household size, in the absence of hired labour, rather than the hiring of labour responding to a fixed landholding. It is certainly different from the more recent standard neoclassical farming household model. This has the 'recursive' property that consumption and labour-supply decisions can be derived from production decisions alone. In particular, labour supply is not restricted to the household's labour force (Singh *et al.* 1986: 7).

Is Chayanov therefore best forgotten, as some would argue? Again, the issue is one of the underlying land and labour institutions, and the degree to which wage labour is available as an input. There are many different accounts of the conditions under which this is so, but a recent influential attempt to provide a comprehensive account of these institutions under different conditions has been made by Hans Binswanger and others. This account is not in fact comprehensive, since its basic dynamic is population growth, and thus it abstracts from other processes of historical change, including, *inter alia*, colonial pressures to create labour markets through taxation and, in parts of Africa, the enclosure of large areas of land by settlers or rich farmers. However, it shows in quite a rigorous way, using ideas of risk and incomplete markets, the continuing relevance of some of Chayanov's ideas for land-abundant agrarian economies.

Household Economy in the Land Abundant Tropics

The overall approach taken by Binswanger and his associates is to construct a general model of agricultural economies, based on decision-making under uncertainty and incorporating problems of incomplete information, and then to apply it to particular cases, such as a land-scarce or land-abundant economy. Binswanger and McIntire (1987) in particular 'analyze the special case of land abundance, simple technology and high transport costs—conditions still found in many parts of sub-Saharan Africa' (p. 74).

The basis of their 'sub-Saharan Africa' model is that, because land is abundant, it has no sales price. They also assume that households have land-use rights in a way similar to that conceived by Chayanov in communal repartitioning. A third relevant assumption is that technology is relatively simple, so that economies of scale in production are limited (Binswanger and McIntire 1987: 75–6). The availability of land implies the absence of a landless class, unlike Hart's case of Java. This in turn means that there is practically no hiring or exchanging of labour in the peak agricultural seasons, since the synchronicity of the crop cycle means that everyone wants to harvest their own crops at the same time.

A direct consequence of these two facets of the land-abundant economy is that 'cultivated area per working household member is largely invariant to household size or wealth' (Binswanger and McIntire 1987: 77). The area cultivated per worker is limited by diminishing returns to labour. Given little variation across households in technology, a corollary of this is Chayanov's hypothesis that cultivated area per household will be determined by the number of workers in the household.

The question that Binswanger and McIntire then raise, which is implicit in Hull's critique, and absent in Chayanov's model, is: what determines household size and composition? For Chayanov, the peasant household was, in the end, a family household, and its size and composition was determined by the life cycle of the family group. In turn, he takes the family as given. Binswanger and McIntire, however, raise the question of why it is advantageous to produce and consume in groups (households). The first reason, they argue, is gains from specialization of various tasks. According to their model, 'these gains exist because of age and sex-specific differences in aptitude, strength, knowledge and experience' (Binswanger and McIntire 1987: 81). While this seems an extremely ahistorical view of the age and sex division of labour, it is close to the complex cooperation argument of Chayanov.

Two further gains exist in having large families, and form the basis for proposing that both horizontal and vertical extended family households will form in these economies. One is in the spreading of risk, and the other is in the older generation exchanging access to capital for the younger generation's cheap labour (Binswanger and McIntire 1987: 82).[2] As a result, young adults in vertically extended households have a greater incentive to remain in households where the head is wealthy. The heads of non-vertically extended households are thus poorer.

However, there are limits to household extension. While a larger household spread risks, it also spreads the pay-off, or insurance against risks, further. Moreover, larger households have to share output between a larger number of people, so that each receives a smaller share, leading to incentive problems. The management of larger households also becomes more difficult.

These are arguments about sharing production rather than residence. Binswanger and McIntire argue that co-residence occurs when larger households experience economies of scale in housework, and when co-residence improves information flows between people, and thus avoids the problem of 'moral hazard', allowing co-residents to 'insure' each other (Binswanger and McIntire 1987: 84).

To summarize the arguments of Binswanger and McIntire, in land-abundant tropical economies, household size and wealth make no difference to per capita production, controlling for age and sex composition. There are, eventually, diseconomies to larger households because of problems of supervision. Household size is partly determined by extension, the incidence of which depends on the wealth of the household head. Age and sex composition matter because of age and sex-specific differences in productivity in certain tasks.

Chayanov vs. Lenin in Tanzania

The nature of land and labour institutions have formed the basis of much subsequent applications of these models to African economies, and Tanzania is

[2] These arguments are derived in part from Meillassoux (1981).

no exception. On one side are those who argue that Tanzania, like most of Africa,[3] is land-abundant, so that land is freely available, usually through some sort of usufructual arrangement. Consequently, it is argued, there is no land market, a limited labour market, and inequality amongst households is, as in Chayanov, driven by the life cycle (Collier *et al.* 1986: 130–2). On the other side are those who hold that these arguments are abstract, or at best unrepresentative of what is going on in the parts of Tanzania where the majority of the population live. These areas are relatively densely populated, with longstanding land and labour markets (van Hekken and van Velsen 1972; Maro 1974; Smith and Sender 1990; Rimmer 1992). Consequently, some of these writers argue that household demography is largely irrelevant to processes of accumulation and labour allocation.

These latter critiques of the inappropriate application of Chayanov to an rural economy are certainly important. However, there are still areas of Tanzania, and indeed other African countries, where land *is not* in short supply, and where labour markets are very limited. These areas may be marginal to the national economy and to likely future dynamics, and contain relatively few people, but they still exist. I will argue in Chapter 6 that this is the case in much of Rufiji, and it was certainly the case in Mng'aru. Moving from a universal certainty that there is no labour and land market to a just as unshakeable belief that these are found everywhere is not useful. Equally, the fact that Chayanov's model is irrelevant to particular empirical cases, such as the Usambaras, while significant, does not mean that it is never relevant.

Beyond the Leninist Critique

Dismissing the Chayanovian model as of no interest on one set of grounds precludes any further consideration of other aspects of it. If we throw the baby out with the bathwater, we cannot examine the baby for defects. Crucial for the present study, there may be other reasons, entirely different from those to do with land and labour markets, why the Chayanovian model is inappropriate. These reasons, however, exist in an intellectual space between the two sides in the debate. They fire salvoes at each other across it, but do not stop to consider what is there. The basic issue at stake is the nature of the life cycle and the household.

Rufiji is a good place to look at these issues precisely because much of the Chayanovian model is applicable. Because it is credible that the influence of the demographic development of households is not immediately swamped by considerations of assets and wage labour in Rufiji, we can start to look at why Chayanov's approach to the household life cycle is so problematic. For what emerges in the second half of this book is that while demographic factors do

[3] See Low (1986) and Shapiro (1990) for applications of Chayanovian ideas to Southern Africa and Zaire respectively.

play a role in household labour allocation, and in economic fortune, they do so not at all in the way that the Chayanovian model indicates.

This conclusion rests on three fundamental findings. First, the complexity of demographic processes in Rufiji—including polygynous marriage, a high rate of divorce and remarriage, sterility and high mortality, and the movement of people, from children to divorced women to elderly relatives' between households—all mean that the household life cycle has only limited meaning. Each life-cycle stage shows impressive variation in household composition within itself, and the life-cycle notion can only account for some of the demographic variation between households.

Ironically, this opens up a possibility which those in the Tanzanian debate have missed, although it has been recognized elsewhere (e.g. Hull 1980). This is that household demography is not purely biologically determined, but is, as noted above, in fact partly *socially* determined. Wealth plays an important role in this social determination. Precisely the processes absent from the biological Chayanovian model—especially polygyny and household extension—can be used by wealthier household heads to enlarge their labour forces. Thus while assets in Rufiji cannot be so easily turned into expanded production through greater inputs and wage labour, they can influence production through the composition and size of the household.

These elements matter because aspects of household structure, although not explained well by the life cycle alone, do affect the labour decisions and burdens of household structure. However, and this is the third point, looking at the behaviour of households alone is to miss almost entirely the point, for far greater variations and responses occur at the level of individuals and subgroups within and between households. The labour patterns of men and women are different, and respond to household characteristics differently.

How relevant is this analysis, given that Rufiji appears increasingly anomalous within the changing Tanzanian economy? Its importance lies in the fact that such dynamics will occur even where Chayanovian assumptions about the rural economy are obviously, even banally irrelevant. Households in all parts of Tanzania have complex demographic cycles, and within broad economic classes, these cycles will have relevance, especially for women's labour. They are likely to be most relevant for the poorest households, precisely because of where these households fit into the labour and land markets.[4] Thus in Smith and Sender's study (1990: 59), we find that the separation or divorce that leads to women heading households in turn forces them into the labour market. In Mng'aru, that is not an option for many women heading households. However, they are still forced to seek sources of cash income in other ways, and this affects their labour allocation differently from women not heading households.

[4] For an excellent example of an analysis of how demographic events determine household fortunes *within given land and labour institutions* in Bangladesh, see Cain (1978).

Gender, Household Composition, and Labour Allocation

The various models discussed here have different approaches to gender. Chayanov does not consider gender, but as Hunt notes (1979: 278), the existence of a rigid sexual division of labour would seriously affect his model: 'In this case one might expect the male : female ratio for productive labour to act as an important determinant of variations in labour allocation and per capita income between households.' Binswanger and colleagues clearly have this in mind when they point to the sex composition of households as having an effect on labour inputs. Shapiro's (1990) study of households in rural Zaire applies this idea by deriving separate relationships between the number of men and women in the household and cultivated area.

However, this conception of gender, as the effect of the sex composition of the household on overall household production, is too abstract and partial. It ignores what has been shown in a variety of settings in Africa—that men and women do not simply have different inputs as household members into an undifferentiated household cultivation, but rather have different specializations in activities, different interests, and different relationships with others both inside and outside the household.[5]

Women and men tend to specialize in different types of crop, with consequences for marketing and income. They also often combine labour in particular tasks on a given crop, so that men may clear land, women plant and weed, men harvest, etc. Thus a sexual division of labour can be task-specific or crop-specific (Whitehead 1981). In Rufiji, we have seen that rice cultivation has become a particularly female crop. The ramifications of this for labour allocation emerge in Chapter 9.

Notions of the household have, of course, developed substantially since Chayanov, and the household of Binswanger and others allows for internal problems of incentives in labour allocation. Problems of the division of product, however, are not discussed, and gender arises only so far as 'sex-specific' skills are considered. The basic problem here is that all members of a household (or production group) are considered to have symmetrical relations with each other. By contrast, studies of gender relations in labour allocation and division of product reveal unequal abilities to mobilize labour and make claims on others, both inside and outside the family. Men can generally make greater claims on women than vice versa. The claims that women can make also vary with their status, in terms of marriage, age, and kinship.

What this implies is that men and women experience household membership (and therefore household composition, wealth, etc.) differently. Their labour inputs should not be considered as contributing to a generalized household cultivation, but rather to specific crops or tasks. Their labour allo-

[5] There is now a huge literature on gender and the household in Africa. Good discussions and overviews can be found in Guyer 1981; Folbre 1986; Evans 1991; and Whitehead 1991.

cations are not the result of natural sex-specific skills,[6] but rather the result of gender- and status-specific claims over others inside and outside the household.

Mng'aru: the Village and the Valley

The remainder of the second part of this book is taken up with an investigation of these issues in a small village, Mng'aru. The village is in the northern part of Rufiji District, about five km. south-east of the end of the tarred road from Dar es Salaam at Kibiti. As described below, Mng'aru lies at the edge of the Magongo Hills and its agricultural system includes rice cultivation. Lying as it does on the cusp of the hill and valley ecologies and farming systems, the village is in one sense an ideal site for research, since the situation there reflects processes occurring over a large part of the district.

Mag'aru is an *ujamaa* village (registered in 1974) with a total population in November 1985 of 573 people. It has declined in size over the last decade, according to censuses taken in 1978 and 1984.

Population of Mng'aru village and number of households

Year	Total population	No. of households
1978	691	156
1984	654	130
1985	573	120

Sources: 1978, 1984—Official village estimates; 1985—Household survey.

Immediately to the west of the village is a prison farm with a population of about 100–200 in total. The economic relationship between the prison and the village is minimal, except that the warders and their families form a market for small-scale trading and for beer. In the village centre in the mid-1980s there was an office of the ruling Chama cha Mapinduzi (CCM) party and the village primary school with adjacent housing for three teachers. Also in this central part is a building housing a maize-milling machine and a paddy-husking machine. These machines, which had an intermittent working history, broke down in the spring of 1986, and were awaiting parts in October. They had been purchased by the village with a loan from the Tanzania Rural Development Bank. Next to the milling machines is the small market place and the tea shop. The other building of note is the village cooperative shop, facing the school.

[6] For a critique of this naturalistic argument see Harris (1981).

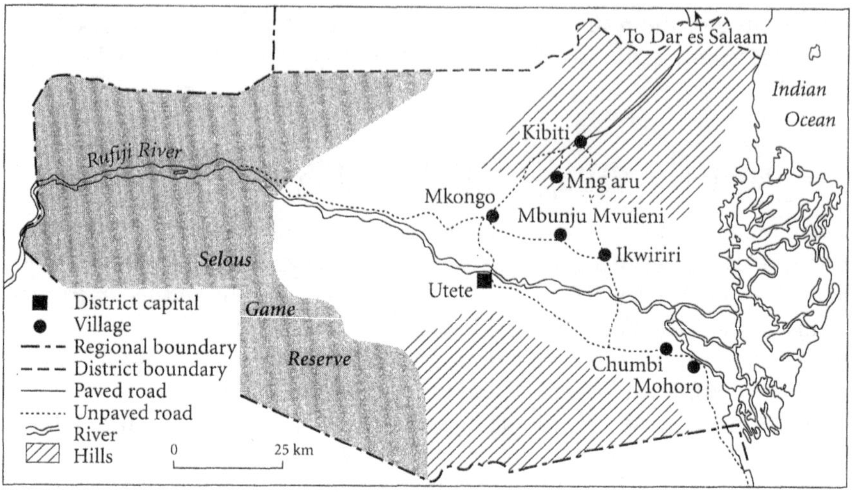

Map 2 *Rufiji District: villages and roads*

The village, in a manner common to the entire coastal area, is divided geographically and genealogically into two parts, around the centre. Strung out northwards along the road to Kibiti is the part known as *ng'ambo*. In this section live some of the longer-established families, but also newcomers, many outsiders to the locality. The middle of the village is the oldest part, and is formed by the houses of the founding lineage (Mtandika), one of whose number was in 1985–6 the CCM Chairman for the Coast Region. The southern part of the village is largely more recent. It was greatly expanded in 1974, when the inhabitants of a small hamlet about two miles away in the valley were moved into the main village. The name of the southern part of the village, *bondeni* (in the valley), thus reflects the origin of its inhabitants.

The whole village lies along a southern-facing spur, Wingayongo Hill, at the edge of the Magongo Hills. Directly below the village to the east is the valley of the Ruhoi River, a tributary of the Rufiji. This is not floodplain, but is formed of heavy, poorly drained clays, and in the *masika* or heavy rains, pools of water remain on the fields for long periods. These 'semi-*mlao*' conditions (Marsland 1938: 56) allow extensive rain-fed rice cultivation. The rice fields spread around the spur of the hill, and lineages have cultivation rights specific to particular sections of the valley. To the east of the village the valley is called *Kopea* and is farmed by families from the *ng'ambo* part of the village, and from the centre. The section of *Kopea* nearest the village is also farmed by the prison. In addition to Mng'aru rice-growers, parts of *Kopea* are also cultivated by people from the surrounding villages (Kibiti, Kimbuga, Ngulakula, Miwaga, and Ikwiriri). Cultivators living locally are often joined periodically by relatives from Dar es Salaam.

To the south of the village, the gradient is much gentler, and the section of the plain at the bottom of the spur is called *Mbongola*. This is farmed by families living in the *bondeni* section, as their original hamlet lay between the *Mbongola* site and the current village. These people also form the greater part of the fishing community in the village, and the main fishing areas lie beyond *Mbongola*. Both the main village and the valley have wells supplying water. The village wells lie along a small valley to the west.

The centre of what is now Mng'aru village was established as a lineage hamlet at some time before 1900 by two members of the central lineage in the village and their families. Somewhat later, a second group joined and intermarried with them. By the 1930s, this site was surrounded on all sides by small lineage hamlets ranging in size from 20 to 80 people at distances of a half to three miles. In 1914 the Germans planned to develop the area for the extraction of sulphur from deposits at the Nyongoni hot springs on the Ruhoi river, about four to five miles south of the village, and from a large outcrop of sulphur-bearing sandstone just outside the village. The British administration took up the plans again in the late 1930s, and built the branch motor road from Kibiti, but further activity was again curtailed by the war. Despite the road connections with Dar es Salaam, transport remained problematic: even in 1942 it was thought that it might be cheaper to transport sulphur to DSM by dhow via Kikale. Commercial interest in the site continued with petroleum exploration in the mid-1950s, when a drilling camp was set up by the sandstone outcrop, but no oil was found.

In 1974, plans for the village were drawn up (as for every other *ujamaa* village), but the current shape of the village has evolved more or less independently of these plans. At this point, the group from *Mbongola* was moved to the south of the village. These lineages still regard themselves as distinct from the longer-standing residents. As noted, they form the vast majority of off-season fishermen and supply the market with fish.

Generally, however, Mng'aru is regarded as a *kijiji cha asili*, i.e. a 'natural' or 'original' village, as distinct from villages wholly created in 1974, such as Rusende or Ikwiriri. Nevertheless, the village has functioned as an entity under Party and government policies. As in other areas along the coast, the concentration of population has meant that tree crops—especially cashews and coconuts—associated with the previous hamlet sites have been abandoned. Since 1974 the government has maintained pressure on the villagers to cultivate collectively—either a food reserve (e.g. cassava, grown in 1984), or a cash crop (in 1986 this was sesame). This policy has often been unpopular, and the acreage to be cultivated was an issue of contention between the local government representative in Kibiti and the villagers at the village annual meeting in 1986. Cultivation of the cash crop was only started after a number of visits and exhortations from the ward secretary.

Other than villagization, the main source of social change in recent years has been in the sphere of education. The educational experience of Mng'aru residents, as for the whole of Rufiji, reflects years of neglect and underdevelopment of services. There are no secondary or special school graduates living in the village. The distribution of current or completed types of education shows three streams or trends. Firstly, the enormous increase in primary education for younger cohorts (below age 30) reflects the universal primary education (UPE) programme started in 1977. Secondly, the adult education programme, active until the early 1980s in Mng'aru, reached the middle cohorts of adults, but far fewer of the older people. Lastly, the colonial primary system (four years of education) apparently became more widespread over time, as more of the younger cohorts (now aged 40–50) received it than of the older cohorts (now aged 60 and over).[7]

Data Collection

Fieldwork was conceived of as an essential part of the methodology of this study. In the Introduction I referred to issues of interpretation as a rationale for fieldwork. However, there are also, of course, strong arguments for undertaking an extended period of fieldwork on grounds of gathering meaningful and better data.[8] One of the strongest of these is that only through an extended stay does one discover the weaknesses and limitations of the information one collects. Here I briefly describe the ways in which data was collected, and outline the main problems. A more thorough account of problems arising from intersubjectivity in survey data collection is given in Lockwood (1992).

Apart from the birth and marriage histories, most of the information was collected by the author, although initially with the help of an interpreter. Apart from the initial questionnaire, all subsequent questionnaires were written during the course of the fieldwork, based on the experience of living in Mng'aru, and on discussions with villagers. This process also led to a change in the method of preparation. The first questionnaire was written in English and translated into Kiswahili, although much of it consisted just of single words or expressions. Subsequent questionnaires were written in Kiswahili, which was in all but a few cases the language of interviewing. All questionnaires were checked by a 'native speaker', although in Tanzania this doesn't necessarily mean Kiswahili is their first language.

The data forming the core of the quantitative analysis were obtained from a series of questionnaire-based interviews in Mng'aru village carried out between October 1985 and the end of September 1986. In addition, a subsidiary survey was carried out in the nearby town of Ikwiriri, and a series of migration interviews in Chumbi and Mohoro near the delta. The surveys are described in the order in which they took place.

1. A preliminary survey of the characteristics of all households (120) in Mng'aru village, including relationships between members, age, sex, educa-

[7] This finding may be due to selection bias, i.e. older people with more education have moved away or died off at a greater rate than those without education, but this seems unlikely, and in any event it cannot be controlled for here.

[8] There is a large literature on the relative strengths and weaknesses of short surveys and appraisals vs. longer periods of fieldwork. For a useful bibliography see Devereux and Hoddinott (1992).

tion, marital status, and tree-crop ownership. This was followed by a section on housing and land-use. These interviews were conducted by myself and Moshi Mokea from October to November 1985. After a preliminary trip to Mng'aru in early October, it was decided to add in a space for information about children currently living in Dar es Salaam, so that people could be selected for migration interviews at a later date.

2. A series of multiple-round interviews on time use for a sample of forty-three households under the jurisdiction of seven ten-cell leaders (*mabalozi*). These leaders were drawn by systematic random sampling, and were asked to select seven households each. This approach was used because it became clear that it would not be possible to obtain the particpation of all the villagers unless the authority of village structures was involved in the sampling. It thus overcame a problem often mentioned by quantitative fieldworkers where people want to know why they were picked or more commonly why not. Not all *balozi* produced seven households, and some of those chosen were thought to be especially problematic in terms of time interviews, mostly very old people living alone. To these were added three female-headed households, since such households were underrepresented in the *mabalozi*'s choices. This was in part due to the interpretation by the *mabalozi* of my request as the production of a list of adult, married men. It is not clear how far this was due to a concept of household held by the *mabalozi*, as opposed to what is expected of *mabalozi* by government and Party directives, given that at this stage I was still regarded as emanating from those directions, or indeed how separate the two possibilities are. The total of forty-six sample households, in a village of 120 ennumerated households, represents a 38 per cent sample. Testing for significant biases in this sample, relative to the total population, the only major factor was that the sample houses contained a slightly higher proportion of younger people. In terms of trees owned, cultivated area, rice growing, and other age indicators, there were no significant differences.

There were three rounds of interviews, although not all individuals were available in each round. The rounds occurred at different points in the annual agricultural cycle. Round 1 was during January, February, and March, covering planting and early weeding of rice, and weeding and harvesting of valley-grown maize; round 2 was during May, June, and July, covering the rice harvest; and round 3 was during September, covering fishing, house repair, craft production, and preparation of the village fields for cassava and *vuli* maize.

In each of these rounds, people were interviewed by myself or Moshi Mokea about their activities on the previous day. In the form of a narrative, they were asked to recount the time of starting and finishing each activity, from the time they woke to the time they went to sleep at night. Activities were not pre-coded, allowing maximum flexibility of classification: effectively, the classification of activities was generated by the respondents themselves.

For the purposes of analysis, twenty-seven different activities were coded. These reflect the wide range of activities which people in Rufiji may take part in at different times of the year. Not all people participate in every activity—in part a reflection of normative divisions of labour specific to sex and age groups.

3. A birth and marriage history for all 130 women aged 15–70 years in Mng'aru. These interviews were carried out by Nyamatimbwa Sultani between February and April 1986. Between May and September 1986, an enlarged birth and marriage history survey was carried out in Ikwiriri, with the interviews being conducted by Mwoshabani Musa Momboka. One hundred and twenty-six women were chosen by random sample taken from households falling under the jurisdiction of nine ten-cell leaders, in turn selected by systematic sampling from three 'villages' (Ikwiriri is a conglomeration comprising nine administrative village units). The questionnaire included a section on family planning designed in cooperation with Walter Mbunda of UMATI (the family-planning association in Tanzania).

4. A series of interviews with previous migrants to Dar es Salaam, and with parents of migrants currently in Dar es Salaam. These included an account of the process of migration, employment, remittances, and return. After conducting thirty-three interviews in Mng'aru in June–July, the migration study was extended in August and September to include interviews in Chumbi and Mohoro. In these two villages, ten-cell leaders were chosen by systematic sampling and all households under those leaders were approached. Of these, ex-migrants and those with migrant children were interviewed.

There are a number of weaknesses in the data which are important for the analysis. The problems that arose tend to be specific to one or other of the surveys. Thus I will deal with each questionnaire in turn.

1. The household survey. The main problem arising here related to age-reporting. Age-reporting generally, especially for older people, was often vague, with digit preferences for 0 and 5. This was countered where possible by direct observation and estimation, and by the use of a local calendar drawn up in conjunction with my main research assistant.[9]

2. Birth and marriage histories. These interviews involved questions about births, infant deaths, and family planning. It was impractical to carry out these interviews myself. I decided to employ female interviewers, who could only be supervised indirectly. A problem analagous to that of age-reporting arose with the reported dates of birth of children, especially those more than a few years before. As a result, only the reported month and year of birth was used, and it is not clear if these are reliable. A different kind of problem related to the omission of infant deaths. It is almost certain that some infant deaths were omitted by mothers who simply mentioned neither the birth nor death of the child. This problem was particularly noticeable in the Ikwiriri survey, where hardly any deaths were noted at all. With an estimated infant mortality rate of 121 per

[9] Age-reporting is notoriously problematic in Africa. The degree to which reported age is influenced by social standing and interaction between interviewer and respondent is pursued in Lockwood (1992), based on a comparison of self-reported age for adult women, and age reported by their husbands and fathers.

1,000 live births for the Coast Region in 1978 (Population Census 1978, viii: 307) it is extremely unlikely that an accurate survey of 126 women would fail to record more than a few deaths. Consequently, only the data from Mng'aru were used in examining patterns of survivorship.

3. Time-use survey. A number of problems arose here. Some of these are inherent in recall data on time-use. The first concerns the accuracy of the period for which an activity was enumerated. Few people wear watches in Rufiji, and the rate of work is not governed by the clock. Rather, timing and duration of activities is generated by needs such as hunger, in the case of cooking, or of weather, as in waiting for a cooler time of day to start cultivation. Further, as elsewhere,[10] in their ordinary descriptions of work of particular tasks, people refer primarily to doing this or that act, not to spending this or that period of time on it.

Beyond this, talking about time is unavoidably structured by both interviewer and interviewee, no matter how much effort is made to avoid this. Thus many periods within which activities were undertaken were described in easy fractions or multiples of hours; 'I farmed (*nililima*) for two hours' or 'I did that for half an hour' were common responses. Some cross-checking using other factors (e.g. distance, for trips to the shamba or well), and other household members is possible, but in many cases the absence of an objective standard means that further probing on such periods is unlikely to be productive.

A second problem is the identification and classification of activities. As mentioned above, activities were not pre-coded, so no preconceptions of the variety or importance of different kinds of activitiy were imposed. However, in the coding stage, various aggregations were made, and this necessarily relected the stress of the study. In this case, I was particularly concerned to differentiate 'domestic' tasks. A major problem, however, emerged as it became clear that for some periods, two activities were being performed which were difficult to allot to separate periods, on the basis of recall data only. One important activity in these cases of 'joint production' was childcare. Since infants and young children require almost constant passive care and minding, and for infants, intermittent but continual breastfeeding, identifying activities such as 'rest' or 'cooking' as purely doing nothing, or only paying attention to the pots is clearly unsatisfactory. 'Childcare' as a category was thus only as reported, i.e. as a consciously noted activity performed with or without other activities. Much childcare beyond this probably lies in the residual 'rest' category.

Given these rather severe drawbacks, it might be asked: why do recall studies of time-use at all? Surely it would be better to do direct stopwatch observation. Recall was used here primarily because of the type of study undertaken—comparing the time-use of people from many different kinds of household, and comparing the time-use of different people within the same household. This requires a larger number of respondents, and data for household members for the same day. Neither of these would be needed in a study

[10] See Pahl's description of similar problems in the Isle of Sheppey (1984: 256).

with few variables or catgories of explanation, nor if household labour profiles were not required. Added to the fact that only two people (myself and an assistant) were available to do this work within the budget of the study, this meant that direct stopwatch study was impracticable. Moreover, direct observation studies have their own set of problems, including the effect of the presence of the observer on the order and duration of tasks done, and the temptation to help the 'object' of study in difficult or onerous tasks.

Where appropriate, biases or specific weaknesses arising from these problems are pointed out in the text.

The remainder of Part II builds up a picture of household demography and its consequences for patterns of labour in four stages. First, the role that household demography might play, as explained above, depends largely on land and labour institutions. These are examined in Chapter 6. In Chapter 7 I examine how accumulation takes place in the absence of large-scale land and labour markets, and its significance for labour allocation. Chapter 8 describes the life cycle and associated aspects of household demography. Finally, in Chapter 9, household demography and patterns of economic activity are brought together in an assessment of the models outlined here, and of the factors which underlie allocations of labour in Mng'aru.

6 Labour and Land in Mng'aru

The importance of demographic factors for household labour allocation and mobility in a rural economy depends crucially on land and labour institutions. Before we can understand how the life cycle and other demographic household features might influence economic activity in Rufiji we must assess (i) the role of wage labour and land acquisition, and (ii) the sexual division of labour. This chapter examines these institutions in Rufiji which form the background to the resulting process of accumulation, analysed in Chapter 7.

The Agricultural System

Rufiji's economy is still fundamentally agricultural, and productive work is therefore dominated by seasonal cycles of tasks. Much reproductive labour, on the other hand, is repeated on a daily basis. The timing and content of seasonal cycles vary within the district, between hill, floodplain, and delta. In this second half of the book, I am most concerned with a specific location—Mng'aru—and so deal here with the pattern of work found there.

Agriculture in Mng'aru can be classified in several ways: hill vs. valley; pure cash crops, pure food crops, and mixed crops; and 'male' vs. 'female' crops. Data on crops grown was available for 117 households (Table 6.1). The staple foods are rice, cassava, maize, and to a lesser extent bananas. The tree crops of cashews and coconuts are grown by about half the households, while a wide range of fruit, vegetables, pulses, and other crops are also grown.

Agricultural activity in Mng'aru is thus marked by a mixed-cultivation strategy. Over 90 per cent of households were recorded as growing five or more different crops in the previous farming year, and nearly half grew eight or more.

Cassava is grown on sandy soil in and near the village, with the burning and clearing of fields for planting taking place in September and October. Planting of cassava and maize also occurs in this period, which is followed by the short or *vuli* rains. Maize is harvested in December through to February, and finger millet (*mtama*), pigeon peas (*mbaazi*), and cow peas (*kunde*) planted after this. Cassava is stored in the field, and can be dug up at any time after about six months have elapsed. Some households do not always cultivate rice every year, but only one household cultivated only rice and valley maize, so the

Table 6.1. *Crops grown in Mng'aru*

Crop	No. of households growing crop	Percentage of households growing crop
Staples		
Cassava	115	98
Maize	100	85
Rice	96	82
Bananas	83	71
Millet	10	9
Tree Crops		
Coconuts	64	55
Cashews	58	50
Oranges	38	32
Fruit		
Pineapples	83	71
Papaya	40	34
Other		
Cow peas	54	46
Sesame	40	34
Pigeon peas	31	26
Okra	26	22

Source: Household survey, Mng'aru 1985.

cassava/maize ridge agriculture is central to the production of food. Thus the digging of cassava and collection of cassava greens (*kisamvu*) is done on an almost daily basis.

The preparation of the rice fields in the valley below Mng'aru starts in October and November, after some rain has fallen to soften the earth. Rice and maize are intersown, and vegetables (such as okra and pumpkin) are sown around the *dungu* to provide a source of *mchuzi* (sauce) during the stay in the rice fields. After planting, the main tasks in the rice fields are weeding and scaring away pests such as birds and monkeys. During this period, through the long or *masika* rains, many of the women live in the valley, with only the men and older children remaining in the village.

Children take over some of the domestic tasks in the village, and play the crucial role of bringing food and implements from the village to the rice fields. Harvesting, threshing, and winnowing the rice take place in June and July, after which the rice is transported back to the village and the 'slack' season begins, roughly from July to September. This is the busy season for weddings, *unyago*, and spirit possession *ngomas*—not only because people have more time and energy, but also because they (especially women) have more money at this time of the year than at any other.

The main cash crops in Mng'aru are tree crops—cashews, coconuts, and citrus fruit—and rice. Cashews require regular tending, and the harvesting of nuts is done during the *vuli* season, with marketing in December. Coconuts are harvested and marketed locally all year round, while citrus fruit are picked and sold locally or transported up to Dar es Salaam in the post-rice harvest season.

In addition to agriculture, extractive and craft activities are important in Rufiji, but do not all follow such a clear seasonal pattern. One of the main extractive activities is charcoal preparation, which is carried on all year round, except during *masika*. The process takes about a month, depending on the number of people involved. Another dry-season extractive activity is fishing, which is mainly done by families living in the *mbongola* section of the village.[1] With the return to the village after the rains and the rice harvest, there is usually a large amount of house repair and rethatching to be done, and more basketry and mat-making takes place. Elsewhere in Rufiji, more time-intensive crafts are usually done more often in the dry season (Havnevik 1983). In Mng'aru the two important crafts are pottery and brewing. There are three kinds of brewing: cashew apple wine (*ulaka*), millet beer (*pombe*, *ugimbi*), and a sugar-based spirit (*gongo*, *pombe ya moshi*, etc.). The first two are seasonal, but the last is distilled whenever sugar is available.

Seasonal labour peaks and food shortages follow the agricultural cycle. Labour peaks occur in November to January with the planting of valley rice and maize and the harvesting of ridge maize and cashews, and again in May to

	Jan.	Feb.	Mar.	Apr.	May	June	July	Aug.	Sept.	Oct.	Nov.	Dec.
									Preparation of fields			
Maize	.... harvest										planting	....
Rice	....	weeding	....	....	...... harvest	....						planting
Peas/okra	planting	....	....	...... harvest								
Cassava	planting	....	....	....	....	....	harvest					
Cashews						weeding	....	....	harvest			
Millet		planting	....	....	....	....	....	harvest				
Sesame		planting	....	....	....	....	harvest					
Labour peaks	*****					************						**********
Food shortages	**********			**************								*******

Fig. 6.1 *Seasonal cycles in Mng'aru*

[1] See Introduction to Part II.

early July with the rice harvest followed closely by the harvesting of sesame, planted as a village crop. There is thus considerable seasonal variation in the time spent in farming. Time-use is discussed in more detail below, but it is worth noting here that the amount of time spent on farming by men in the time-use sample falls from over four hours a day in January to about forty minutes a day in September. For women the figures are from around three hours a day to just over an hour. There is by contrast very little seasonal variation in the time spent in domestic labour.[2]

Food shortages generally precede harvests, falling in October, early November, and especially in April and early May. All these timings are dependent on the rains, and vary from year to year. The agricultural cycle is shown in full in Fig. 6.1.

Gender Divisions of Labour

Normative divisions of labour

Lévi-Strauss (1963: 281) observes that norms are 'conscious models', implying a different level of moral meaning from the merely statistical. However, if the conscious model (or a dominant conscious model) is taken too literally, there may be no consideration of deviant cases, and the existing pattern may be taken as timeless or eternal. As Lévi-Strauss goes on to say, norms function to perpetuate, not to explain. 'Normal' divisions of labour can hence best be understood as rules that people try to avoid breaching—and indeed will go to great lengths to do so.[3] However, since situations do arise where, from necessity, these divisions are breached, they are not as general as they might first appear. Children and unmarried youths are especially flexible with regard to divisions of labour by sex.

Table 6.2 gives an outline of activities differentiated by gender in Mng'aru. These roles were identified partly through observation and partly in discussion with villagers. There are other agricultural and craft activities not covered

[2] Seasonal variation in domestic labour is not significant at the 10 per cent level, whereas time spent in productive labour is. For definitions of these labour categories see below.

[3] For example, a norm for the division of labour in Rufiji is that married men do not cook. Note that such men generally do know the culturally specific process of cooking, since many have lived on their own, or as co-tenants, in Dar es Salaam or elsewhere. Some of the older men also learned some domestic skills from employment in domestic service (Bujra 1987), although these skills may not always be directly applicable in the material and cultural setting of Rufiji. However, what is suitable for the bachelor is not suitable for the married man, since the latter has obtained through marriage the domestic services of his wife (as the marriage ceremonies explicitly demonstrate). In the house in which I was living in Mng'aru, the owner had been left by his wife some weeks before my arrival. In place of his wife, he called upon a female relative, in this case a parallel maternal first cousin, to do his cooking. After a while, she got tired of this, and he had to find another female relative to take the place of the cousin. During the rice harvest, when almost all the women of the village were living in the valley, some 3 km. away, he was forced to cook for the household himself, calling on knowledge gained from his days in Dar es Salaam. This, however, was regarded as an entirely temporary and slightly shaming solution.

Table 6.2. *Normative divisions of labour by gender (adults)*

Task	Male	Female
Agriculture		
Burning and clearing of fields	×	
Preparation of fields	×	×
Planting	×	×
Weeding cassava	×	×
Weeding rice	(×)	×
Guarding crops (day)	(×)	×
Guarding crops (night)	×	(×)
Harvesting rice (cutting)	×	×
Threshing/winnowing rice		×
Digging cassava	(×)	×
Wage labour	×	
Domestic tasks		
Peeling/drying cassava	(×)	×
Pounding		×
Cooking		×
Washing clothes	×	×
Fetching water		×
Fetching firewood	×	×
Childcare	(×)	×
Washing dishes/sweeping		×
Crafts		
Carpentry	×	
Plastering/mortar making	×	
String-bed-making	×	
Basketry	×	×
Mat-making	×	×
Pottery		×
Blacksmith	×	
Carving	×	
Bicycle repair	×	
Extractive activities		
Charcoal	×	(×)
Wood-cutting	×	
Fishing	×	
Construction		
Housebuilding	×	
Building *madungu* for rice cultivation	×	×
Thatching	×	(×)
Marketing		
Local marketing	×	(×)
Formal crop-marketing	×	
Informal crop-marketing	×	×

Note: See also Havnevik (1983: 51–7). Only activities relevant to Mng'aru have been listed here. Other activities, such as skilled crafts and *maandazi/vitumbua* marketing, would be more important in Kibiti, Ikwiriri, and Mohoro.

Sources: Interviews and author's observations.

here which are common to other ecological zones of the district, such as mangrove cutting and coconut oil production in the delta, so that this should not be treated as a complete system. However, it comprises the most common and important day-to-day activities, outside of ceremonial, religious, and ritual practice, performed in Mng'aru.

Within this system, activities are defined as either exclusively male or female (e.g. fetching water is women's work) or as not specifically gendered (e.g. fetching firewood). Where activities are indicated in brackets, this means that the activity is primarily within the domain of the other gender, but in certain circumstances can legitimately be performed by the gender in question, or it means that it is principally in the domain of the other gender but not exclusively. Thus for example, childcare is almost always the responsibility of women (or older children), but in the evening, while the woman (or women) of the house is (are) cooking, it is possible to find men minding the younger children. Furthermore, this is not seen as a breaching of the division of tasks. In the case of an activity such as charcoal preparation, while this is not defined as an exclusively male undertaking, it is so often performed by men, rather than by women, that it is worth distinguishing from more equally non-gendered tasks such as field preparation.

Broadly speaking, the normative adult gender division of labour is that women do tasks directly concerned with the daily running of the household, men do more crafts, extractive activities, and marketing, and both do agricultural work. In the latter, men specialize more in the 'heavier' tasks such as field clearing, and women in the 'lighter' tasks such as guarding the crops from birds and monkeys, and winnowing, but both sexes participate in a wide range of agricultural processes. In general, in agriculture, a substantial degree of complexity and coordination is involved between people, and the gender division of labour reflects this. For example, although rice cultivation can be an individual undertaking, cooperation following the lines of the division of labour make possible what each individual separately might not have been able to do. Thus a young man may clear a new *shamba*, his grandmother guard it, both of them harvest the rice, and his grandmother and any other female relatives thresh and winnow.

Observed divisions of labour

Quantitative measures of the reported actual sexual division of labour are shown in Table 6.3. The data in this table are from the time budget survey which is described in the Introduction to Part II. Data are averaged over seasons. The parallels with the normative division of labour in Table 6.2 are clear. Men and women participate in agricultural labour on an almost equal basis, but some men participate in a far wider range of productive activities. By contrast, men do hardly any domestic work, while women spend on average over five hours a day in reproductive tasks. The variation in their time spent on cooking, food preparation, and collecting water is relatively low, showing that most women do these things on most days.

Table 6.3. *Time spent on tasks by sex (adults aged 16+): means and standard deviations* (minutes)

Task	Men		Women	
	Mean	S.D.	Mean	S.D.
Production	267	207	190	173
Farming	198	201	169	161
Guarding crops	15	55	16	77
Charcoal	13	79	3	33
Wage labour	13	58	0	0
Fishing	12	49	0	0
Carpentry	4	31	0	0
Trading	11	71	1	16
Domestic tasks	30	95	325	183
Childcare	0	0	31	93
Cooking	11	41	138	92
Firewood collection	4	17	8	23
Food prep.	12	52	71	86
Water collection	2	12	60	49
Washing dishes	1	5	18	28
Crafts	42	103	11	47
Crafts	23	74	11	47
House-building	19	68	1	1
Other	127	157	44	90
Travel	37	114	3	31
Village/co-op work	22	65	8	47
Travel to *shamba*	68	103	34	70
N	101		122	

Source: Time-use surveys, Mng'aru, 1986.

Types of Labour

Thus far, 'labour' has been differentiated in terms of tasks. Another way of looking at divisions of labour is to distinguish between different forms of work or between different sources of labour in the production of goods and services. Pahl gives a detailed account of these divisions in a contemporary English community based on a particular typology of kinds of work (Pahl 1984: 123–5). This typology differentiates work according to the context in which it is done, regardless of the task itself. Thus he distinguishes wage work, self-employed petty commodity production—both officially registered and in the shadow economy—employment by the state, social reproduction under capitalist and patriarchal relations (and not under those relations), and other work contributing to the survival and solidarity of the group. Developing an analogous classification of labour for Rufiji, where most labour is far less dominated directly by state or capital, requires slightly different categories. In particular, for a village like Mng'aru, the relative unimportance of wage labour (see below) means that the source of labour is almost always 'family' labour. A more important distinction lies in with and for whom the work is performed. This is because clear distinctions are made in Rufiji between different categories of responsibility.

First, there is the responsibility of both men and women to contribute money and labour to the common family pool. These duties are mostly defined in terms of food. Thus there is a general expectation that men should provide cash for those items of food, such as fish, salt, dried beans, and some vegetables, that need to be bought in the market place. Indeed, the actual buying of such food is usually done by men. Both men and women, but more centrally women, are expected to provide labour for crops which will be eaten by the family as a group. Such 'family labour' is, in villages on or near the valley terraces such as Ikwiriri, Mkongo, or Mng'aru, associated with specific crops, such as cassava. This is contrasted with rice, the cultivation of which is more individual, as is the control of the rice harvested. Also included in this category of labour is much of what is also called domestic labour—the collection of water, firewood, cooking, and food processing.

A second class is where a person is perceived as responsible for providing goods or services to another particular person rather than to the family as a whole. Taxation for plural wives in the 1920s was possibly of this type: certainly the view of the colonial administration was that men were responsible for paying their wives' taxes (TNA 1733/18: 105). This issue reappeared in 1986 with the development levy (a poll tax). Initial confusion about whether or not the tax applied to women gave rise to a debate about who should, and who was able, to pay. Other examples would include the responsibility of a father to provide school uniforms and equipment for his children; and the very wide range of services, from sexual favour to cooking, that a woman contracts to provide for her husband in Islamic marriage.

Lastly, there is a class of labour or expenditure which it is the responsibility of the individual to provide for himself or herself. These roles start at as young an age as possible: by their early teens, children of both sexes are expected to provide part or all of the cost of their clothing. Often, girls do this by selling rice that they have grown, and boys through fishing or casual piece-rate labour. The individual status of responsibility for clothing extends to the washing of clothes: this is one 'domestic' task that women do not do for their husbands or families. Expenditures of this sort are thus not normally expected by anyone of anyone else, which is why they can attain the status of a gift, as is the case of clothing, apart from the obvious reason that clothing is expensive. Similarly, this is why clothing and other items of 'individual' expenditure form the basis of a person's inalienable property in marriage settlements. Such expenditures are also associated with certain kinds of labour, in the sense that the proceeds of certain activities cannot legitimately be claimed by the family pool, or by another, although they may be given voluntarily. Such activities include: for both sexes, part of the proceeds of rice cultivation; for women, brewing or making and selling *maandazi* etc.; for men, charcoal production, and part of the proceeds of fishing. Such labour is reflected in the organization of (especially rice) cultivation (see below).

This categorization of labour and money by 'responsibility' of expenditure has implications for describing the division of labour. It means that a concept such as the gender division of labour cannot be applied directly to tasks such as 'collecting water from the well'. Although collecting water is *generally* described as 'women's work', i.e. meaning the task performed as part of a woman's responsibility to the family, or to her husband, men will also carry water, either as wage labour, or if needed for a project on their own account, such as the distillation of *gongo*, or the washing of their own clothes. They would not, legitimately, be able to get a woman to perform this task for them in these circumstances. Divisions of labour must therefore be defined not only in terms of tasks, but as tasks done for oneself, for another, or for the family. This is precisely the point made by Pahl, in his extended example of ironing a shirt (Pahl 1984: 123–4).

Types of labour arise out of the fact that neither whole (nuclear) families nor residential households in Rufiji are productive units, either in the sense that everyone actually works together, or that their activities are coordinated under a single rubric. It is in this sense, rather than in issues of land supply and wage labour, that Chayanov's model of the peasant household is not directly applicable.

In three important ways, labour is organized along other lines. First, individuals sometimes work alone, directing their own work effort, *on their own fields*. Secondly, people within residential households form 'subgroups' to work together, sometimes, but not always, on *family plots*. Thirdly, there is cooperation between members of different residential households. This is most visible in certain activities, such as charcoal burning, and rice harvesting, and threshing. Cooperation in groups *within* households is important for the analysis of dependency and labour attempted below. Some indication of its pattern is given in Tables 6.4 and 6.5. These tables are derived from the time-use surveys in Mng'aru. They show the responses to questions about with and for whom particular kinds of work were done. The numbers refer to the frequency of cooperation or service.

The main patterns shown in the tables are fairly clear. Women and girls display a far higher level of cooperation than do men and boys, over a greater range of tasks. Men's main cooperation is in farming with their wives, but the latter coordinate their energies more widely with female relatives, especially in food preparation and cooking. Women and girls cooperate more with each other, in same sex groups, and in domestic work.

Setting these categories down on paper gives them a formality and completeness of expression that is not present in reality. Although they constitute a 'moral economy', and evoke strong feelings about what is right and wrong, they are clearly not (if they are ever) fully observed. This implies both conflicts

Table 6.4. *Frequency of tasks performed with or for another: adults*

Activity	Women aged over 20 years					Men aged over 20 years				
Done for/with	C	Z	Co-W	H	OFR	C	W	OR	Emp	Uj
Domestic	24	10	16	0	7	1	0	0	0	0
Agricultural	4	3	4	6	6	2	18	3	2	3
Other economic						0	0	5	2	0

Note: C = children; W = wife/ves; Emp = employer; OR = other relative; Uj = working with other villagers on ujamaa plots; Z = sister; co-W = co-wife; H = husband; OFR = other female relative.

Source: Assistance survey, Mng'aru, 1986.

Table 6.5. *Frequency of tasks performed with or for another: children*

Activity	Girls aged under 20 years					Boys aged under 20 years					
Done for/with	M	Z	B	OFR	Friend	M	Z	B	Sib	F	Emp
Domestic	22	39	3	11	3	3	1	5	9	0	0
Agricultural	6	8	4	1	0	3	2	5	6	5	5

Note: M = mother; Sib = unspecified sibling (*ndugu*); Z = sister; F = father; B = brother; Emp = employer; OFR = other female relative.

Source: Assistance survey, Mng'aru, 1986.

and the possible decline or change of institutions for allocating labour and product, as the stresses on these principles change over time. A major site of conflict was, as described in Chapter 5, responsibilities for providing labour to an apparently common pool. The use of this principle by men to appropriate the labour of wives seems to have been an attempt, in the 1920s and 1930s, by richer men to circumvent the lack of a labour market during the expansion of cotton and rice acreages and sales (TNA 1733/18: 105; Telford 1929: 26). Such struggles, both over the relative time spent on 'individual' and 'family' crops, and over the blatant appropriation of women's rice by their husbands, clearly continue (Swantz 1985: 39–40).

The data above under-record the importance of extra-familial labour working parties for certain, specialized activities. While there was general agreement in Mng'aru that food and beer working parties were more common in the past than now, erosion of this organizational form is uneven. Working parties were usually single-sex, and both male and female parties were taken from descent groups. However, while male extra-familial cooperation has much declined, and persists now mostly in a different form in charcoal preparation, female cooperation remains important in the harvesting and threshing of rice—symbolically central and still economically significant in Rufiji life. Such labour is done collectively by women belonging to a given patrilineage by birth or by marriage. They rotate around the plots, harvesting and threshing the rice of each member by turn. By contrast, communal labour in charcoal preparation, both male and female, is not necessarily organized along kin lines at all, and is based on payment rather than reciprocation, even though the payment may be in beer or a share of the charcoal.

Land and Wage Labour

We now turn to wage labour.[4] The initially most striking aspect of the labour market in Rufiji is that it is small. This is the case not only currently, or after the Arusha Declaration, but has historically been so. Wage labour in agriculture became an issue in periods of attempted intensification of cultivation. On the eve of the 1930s, which saw a large, state-run programme of increasing cotton and other crop output, Telford noted that the idea of employing direct wage labour was quite new to the district, and was not taken up to any great extent (Telford 1929: 37). Such 'Grow More Crops' campaigns were repeated after the war, and certain farmers, identified as 'progressive', were encouraged to hire labour (Coulson 1978: 78–9). Within Rufiji, this period of the 1950s and 1960s may have seen the widest spread of wage labour in agriculture, especially in the downstream areas. Nevertheless, systematically hiring labour on a large scale was essentially innovative behaviour, and like other innovative practices in the 1950s and 1960s, led to hostility and resentment within these communities. This reaction to the nascent shift from ascribed status to acquired status through accumulating surplus led to fear of and accusations of witchcraft, which were powerful stimulants to seeking opportunities elsewhere. People were cursed for being able to buy a bicycle, or to put *mabati* roofing on their houses. Such conditions not only blocked the development of labour-hiring practices within the district, but also encouraged successful migrants to invest in Dar es Salaam, or even to remain there permanently. By the time that the communities had been transformed (and transported) by villagization, this opposition to large-scale labour hiring had become (at least nominally) official policy through the Arusha Declaration. In his 1974 survey of Rufiji, Yoshida found that wage labour provided on average only 10 per cent of household income in the downstream areas.[5]

[4] In Mng'aru, most wage labour was piece-rate labour, i.e. a lump sum payment for the completion of an agreed job, rather than time rate.

[5] Cited in Bantje (1979: 10).

In Mng'aru in 1985–6, wage labour was rare. Tables 6.4 and 6.5 show the low frequency of males reporting that they did labour for an employer. There are only ten occasions out of over a hundred days of observations. Equally, only thirteen out of the more than 150 adult men in the village gave wage labour as a secondary occupation. None gave it as a primary occupation—everyone identified themselves as a farmer.

Apart from the perceived threat to political balance, four factors underlie the absence of a labour market and investment in capitalist farming in Rufiji. One is to do with land, two are connected with the cropping system, and the last is an outcome of the history of migration from Rufiji.

As in the whole of Tanzania, land in Rufiji was officially inalienable from the nation. In practice, land is so plentiful in the district—population density in 1978 was 10.1 persons per square mile, according to the census—that the *de facto* land market emerging elsewhere is more or less absent in Rufiji. Under such conditions, the important aspect of land allocation is access to land, or usufruct rights, rather than ownership. As in many systems along the coast,[6] usufruct rights in Rufiji are accorded by membership of a kin group—here *ukoo*, the patrilineal descent group. Membership of this group is significant in other matters, including the coordination of bridewealth payment, and of ritual and its expenses. *Ukoo* is thus a principle of authority which cuts across the official structures of village council, ten-cell leaders, etc. In some coastal descent systems, e.g. northern Mafia, the principle of cognatic descent extends to land rights. In Rufiji, however, while matrilineal kin are the source of some properties (possession by certain *mashetani* for instance), land rights are accorded by membership of the agnatic group only.

Thus every person is entitled to access to land, either by direct group membership, or for some women through their husbands. This has two corollaries. First, although there are inequalities between and within *ukoo* of quantity and quality of land, these are relatively small. As we shall see below, the distribution of land used in Mng'aru is relatively egalitarian, and this includes land under tree crops, which skews the distribution. In Telford's 1929 survey, the largest area cultivated was 8.3 acres, and this was in a household with four adults. All but two of the households he surveyed farmed less than five acres (Telford 1929: 27). According to figures obtained from the agricultural officer for the Mohoro Division, average acreages cultivated per household for Chumbi and Mohoro in 1985–6 was just below three. Other sources within Chumbi village put the average farmed at about four to six acres. The slightly larger acreages farmed downstream may reflect the greater purchase of tractor-ploughing services there; one person in Chumbi was farming thirty acres. Generally, however, the lack of a market in land makes it necessary for those who use large tracts of land to provide an account

[6] See Caplan (1982).

of their activities either to the *ukoo*, or, eventually, to the village and party authorities.

The second point, merely the obverse of the first, is that no one is forced into relying exclusively on the sale of their labour power through lack of land: there is no landless class of labourers. While control over, or access to, land as a means of production through kin institutions is not as secure as individual private ownership, and such control and access is often mediated by others, all have recourse in the end to the principle of access, which is widely accepted.

A second factor constraining the development of a large labour market is the seasonally bunched nature of labour demand in agriculture. This is a feature accentuated in the floodplain agricultural system, where the rice harvest and *mlau* planting coincide (Bantje 1979: fig. 1), but it is also present in the hills and delta. In 1934, for instance, attempts to establish commercial mangrove bark collection by the Liverpool Uganda Company foundered on the clash between their labour needs and the annual movement of people away from the delta to the floodplain to plant rice (TNA 61/3/IX/D).

The importance of the seasonality of certain labour demand peaks arises out of the fact that all adults (effectively all married adults) have their own land to work. This means that, for example, in the few days of peak activity during the rice harvest, they cannot cut their own rice and that of others for wages at the same time. In these circumstances, it is not surprising that only those without their own *shamba*, i.e. young unmarried men, form the casual labour supply.

The third factor constraining the development of capitalist farming is the basic uncertainty arising from flood and rain patterns. This is stressed in the work of Bantje, and is constantly referred to by local government workers in the district, as well as by the farmers themselves. In the 1960s, control of the valley ecology to allow systematic investment in farming was supposedly one of the motives behind plans to construct a dam at Steigler's Gorge. However, large-scale farming has been absent from Rufiji until 1988, when an Iranian-run project was instigated to grown irrigated rice west of Ikwiriri. The scheme was behind schedule, and was not ready for the 1988 season. In fear of the effects of flooding, rice was planted quite high on the valley. However, with the highest flood since 1974 occurring in 1989, much of the crop was still lost. The project's problems are confounded by the land factor: there is local suspicion of a scheme which is perceived as a threat to rights over the best land.[7]

A fourth factor was labour migration to Dar es Salaam (see Chapter 4). The growth of labour migration from Rufiji, which was considerable after the Second World War, both arose out of the absence of large-scale acceptable wage-labour opportunities in the district, and contributed to the damping down of wage labour.

[7] Paul Smithson, personal communication, 24 July 1989.

As a consequence of the unviability of large-scale or capitalist agriculture in Rufiji, most accumulation is through trade. Rufiji's merchant class has a long history, dating back (as elsewhere in Tanzania) to the trade in slaves, ivory, food, and other products with Zanzibar and Kilwa. It has also been delineated ethnically, with Asians and Arabs dominating trade until (and even after) Independence. They enjoyed the protection of the Germans under Rechenburg, but later came under pressure from the British administration, who saw them as disrupting extraction by the colonial state.[8] During the Second World War, food marketing was centralized under government control, but was privatized again after the war up to the late 1950s (TNA 1943; Bryceson 1987). This was a good period for the merchants, who maintained their shops after Independence, and diversified into transport and tractor-ploughing services.[9] The principal activities of traders in Mohoro and the lower river valley now involve the leasing of tractors and other vehicles, operating shops, and transporting. While some made their initial money through farming, or from coconut plantations, they did not plough back the proceeds to any great extent, preferring to use them for other ventures.[10]

Conclusion

In certain key features, the economy of Rufiji matches the Chayanovian model, and even more so the Binswanger model. The supply of land is flexible, and access to it through *ukoo* or individual usufruct is a relatively close approximation to 'communal repartitioning', in that it can respond to the life cycle of the household. The lack of alienability of land means that there is no land-accumulating class, and no complementary landless class. Almost everyone farms, and all farm roughly the same crops, so that labour peaks come together, and wage labour is not available at peak periods, except for young unmarried men without their own land. The lack of wage labour and the risky nature of farming also inhibit investment in farming, especially in the potentially rich floodplain area. In Mng'aru, farming technology is largely uniform for everyone. All of these factors mean that there are serious limits to the degree which richer farmers can increase their wealth through employing labour. Differentiation is hampered by a lack of convertibility of capital, from money into labour.

The more important divisions of labour occur within households, especially those between men and women. Here, the Chayanovian model breaks down, as it is clear that the allocation of labour between crops and between tasks is not based simply on the size and age composition of the household. Equally, examination of labour roles or types of labour in Mng'aru shown that the notion of the household as a common labouring and consuming unit, present

[8] See Ch. 4.
[9] This is a familiar pattern in a rentier economy—see Mamdani (1987).
[10] See the case-studies in Lockwood (1989*b*: 308–9).

in the Binswanger model, is not applicable. Work and expenditure are not homogeneous, but rather are differentiated according to areas of responsibility. Further, some tasks are taken on not by the household as a whole, but by subgroups within the household, or sometimes by individuals working with individuals from other households.

7 Inequality and Accumulation in Mng'aru

Rufiji is a poor part of a poor country, and for most people the ceiling on accumulation has been low. A major conclusion in the previous chapter was that accumulation through investment in farming and the employment of wage labour are rare. There are a few individuals, mostly traders, who stand out as wealthy men and women in the district. These people command control over considerable productive assets, including tractors, lorries, and houses, as well as large stockpiles of food and other agricultural produce. They are generally found in the larger centres, of Utete, Mkongo, Ikwiriri, and Mohoro. However, they are conspicuously absent in Mng'aru, where no-one owns a vehicle. For the majority of the population then, inequality consists in contrasts in the number of personal assets and cashew and coconut trees owned. In this chapter I examine patterns of inequality in Mng'aru, and the processes of accumulation which lie behind them. The purpose of the chapter is twofold. First, to understand how accumulation works, in the absence of wage labour, and therefore relying largely on family labour. Second, to investigate the degree to which wealth, as opposed to demographic factors, may affect economic activity in Mng'aru.

Land

As described above, land in Mng'aru is administered loosely by *ukoo* kin groups, with a fair amount of individual initiative. Under this system, it is difficult for individuals to appropriate large concentrated areas of land. From Table 7.1, showing the distribution of plot sizes, it is clear that most farming on individual plots is done on a small scale.

Figure 7.1 shows the Lorenz curve for the distribution of land per adult among households. Although this distribution is affected by tree ownership, it shows that land access, controlling for household size, is not particularly unequal. The distribution has a Gini coefficient of 0.314.[1]

The distribution of land amongst households is, however, complicated by interrelationships between levels of control of resources. Land in Mng'aru is

[1] The Gini coefficient focuses attention on inequality in the mid-range of the distribution, but is useful for comparability because of its wide application. The coefficient here is low: for example, that for pre-tax *income* in OECD countries for the period 1967–72 averaged 0.366, while that for Japan—noted for its equality of distribution—in 1969 was 0.316 (Kuznets 1988: 512).

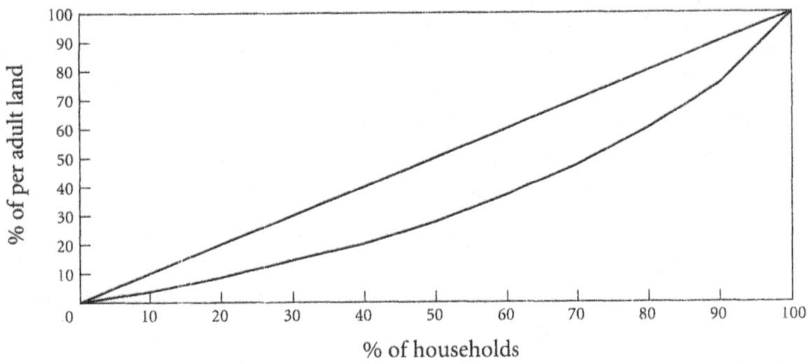

Fig. 7.1 *Per adult land distribution*

Table 7.1. *Plot size distribution*

Acreage	No. of plots	Percentage of plots	Percentage of total land
<1	33	11.3	3.2
1–2	148	50.9	35.2
2–3	75	25.8	33.2
3–5	29	10.0	20.0
>5	6	2.1	8.4

Source: Household survey, Mng'aru, 1985.

still readily available, although the clearing of new land involves a large initial labour input. Tree crops, in contrast to land, are owned by individuals; mostly, as we shall see, by (male) household heads. Household wealth in turn is then largely related to the wealth of those household heads.

Tree Ownership

Tree crops are a major form of productive investment in Mng'aru. Not only do they bear fruit over a long period, but they are a store of wealth, since they can be sold and bought, and indeed inherited. Cashews were introduced to Mng'aru in the 1950s by one of the leading families in the village, and were particularly important during the 1960s and 1970s. However, falling prices, villagization, and disease have led to their decline (Ellis 1980). Coconuts are a longer-standing part of the Rufiji economy. On the coast, where they are grown in large plantations, they can form the basis for considerable wealth. In a place like Mng'aru, they are planted on a smaller scale, but are still a key resource.

Taking all adult men (aged 16 and over) in the village, the distribution of tree ownership is highly unequal; over half the men in Mng'aru owned no cashew trees at all, while the figure for coconuts is 45 per cent. When looking at the distribution of trees amongst only those men with trees, the inequality is still pronounced, as the Lorenz curves in Fig. 7.2 show. The Gini coefficients (amongst owners) for cashews is 0.45, and that for coconuts is 0.5022.

No similar curve for women is given because their ownership of trees is confined literally to a handful of older widows. Only 4 per cent of women in Mng'aru owned any cashews, while coconuts were owned by 6 per cent. Even these women had relatively few trees.

The processes by which men acquire tree crops may be seen in some of the associations between tree ownership and various characteristics. A preliminary point is that tree accumulation is almost exclusively the activity of married men, and therefore largely household heads. All but two of the forty-three unmarried men aged 16 and over in Mng'aru had no cashews; and thirty-nine of them had no coconuts.

Old men have more trees than young men (Table 7.2). The top six men in both cashews and coconuts distributions, i.e. the owners of 200 or more cashews, or fifty or more coconuts, are all but one aged over 65.

These links between tree accumulation and age reflect three distinct processes. First, specifically for cashews, older men tend to have invested in cashews more than younger men because price and disease factors have made them less attractive since the mid-1970s. Second, tree accumulation takes time. Typically men will build up tree holdings incrementally over a large number of years. Lastly, holdings are partially influenced by inheritance, and older men are obviously more likely to have inherited trees.

Tree ownership is also significantly associated with migration to Dar es Salaam in the past. Ex-migrants have more trees, especially coconuts, than non-ex-migrants (Table 7.3).

The effects of education on tree accumulation are difficult to discern, since the central contrast (between those with and those without modern primary education) is closely associated with age. Adult men with primary education

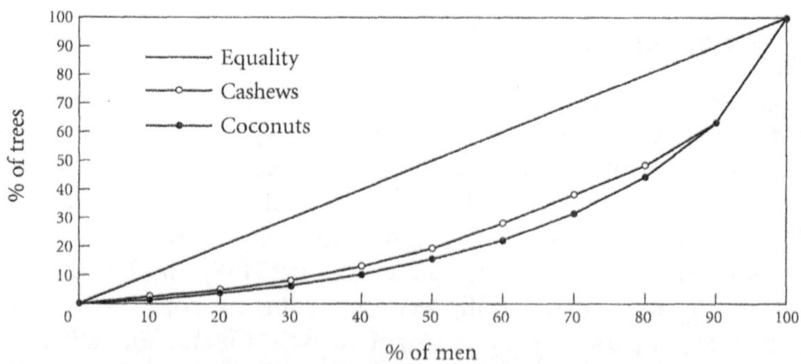

Fig. 7.2 *Distribution of male tree-crop ownership*

Table 7.2. *Distribution of tree ownership by age group (percentages in brackets)*

Age group	Cashews			Coconuts		
	0	1–50	>50	0	1–10	>10
<30	45 (88.2)	6 (11.8)	0 (0.0)	44 (86.3)	5 (9.8)	2 (3.9)
30–50	20 (47.6)	14 (33.3)	8 (19.1)	11 (26.2)	20 (47.6)	11 (26.2)
50–70	7 (25.9)	8 (29.6)	12 (44.4)	1 (3.7)	12 (44.4)	14 (51.9)
>70	8 (30.8)	6 (23.1)	12 (46.2)	10 (38.5)	7 (26.9)	9 (34.6)
Chi-square 47.398, 6 d.f., $P < 0.001$				64.19, 6 d.f., $P < 0.001$		

Source: Household survey, Mng'aru, 1985.

Table 7.3. *Distribution of tree ownership by ex-migrant status*

Previous migration to Dar es Salaam	Cashews			Coconuts		
	0	1–50	>50	0	1–10	>10
No	73 (58.8)	26 (21.0)	25 (20.2)	64 (51.6)	35 (28.2)	25 (20.1)
Yes	7 (31.8)	8 (36.4)	7 (31.8)	2 (9.1)	9 (40.9)	11 (50.0)
Chi-square 5.556, 2 d.f., $P < 0.1$				15.2, 2 d.f., $P < 0.001$		

Source: Household survey, Mng'aru, 1985.

are more likely to have no cashews than those with no education (84 as against 38 per cent). The figures for coconuts are 80 per cent as opposed to 36 per cent. Twenty-one older men received primary education in the late colonial period. Compared to men with no education, these men own fewer cashews, but more coconuts.

Educated men are of course more likely to migrate, so that age, migration, and education (and marriage) are associated factors. To investigate whether all four have independent effects on tree ownership, a multivariate test of significance was carried out, Migration, education, and marital status are significant at the 5 per cent level for coconut ownership, but migration and marital status drop out as insignificant for cashew ownership.

What emerges is a picture of distinct accumulation strategies. Educated men tend to migrate, return, and invest in coconuts, whereas uneducated men have taken more to cashews. The top 5 per cent of the cashew-owning distribution (200 trees or more) contains no ex-migrants and only one man under 65. This is in a sense surprising, since cashews were a new crop in the 1960s, whereas coconuts are of long-standing along the coast. However, the planting of coconuts is also associated with the establishment of a home, and is seen as a long-term investment. They may be especially attractive to migrants who return after a period of city life and wish to marry and establish themselves as 'proper' villagers. The largest holding of coconut palms, of some one hundred trees, belongs to a 32-year-old ex-migrant who has had modern primary education. A final point concerns kinship. The kin groups or *ukoo* in Mng'aru could be divided into larger, well-established groups and smaller, more peripheral groups, often of relative newcomers. Households in the former group own significantly more coconuts than those in the latter group. This factor may work through inheritance, but it may also be that the lines of assistance and information which flow through kin groups when, for instance, raising money for marriage payments, also helps younger men in the *ukoo* to accumulate trees.

Housing and Personal Assets

Richer[2] men in Mng'aru may spend money not only on tree crops, but also or instead on housing and items of personal wealth. Various indicators of such investment were gathered.

Housing costs can vary substantially, from being virtually free if the householder builds for himself and collects all materials locally, up to those who claimed to have spent Tsh. 10,000 on materials and labour. Roofing was divided into three categories: *nyasi* or grass thatching; *makuti* or palm thatching; and *mabati* or tin sheets. These were given ascending scores. Wall quality was divided similarly into four categories: *nyasi*, *makuti*, *udongo* or mud and sticks, and plastered. This last category, requiring considerable expense on paying a specialist plasterer, applied to only six houses, or 5 per cent of the village. Tin roofing, the other high-cost category, was found in fourteen out of 120 cases. The walls and roofing indices were added together to give an overall housing score, ranging from a minimum of two (*nyasi* walls and roofs) to a maximum of seven (plastered walls and tin roof).

Added to these housing scores were personal assets or items, comprising radios, watches or clocks, bicycles, and wooden beds. These items represent significant expenditure, and are not part of craft output in the district. They are assets in the sense that they are a store of wealth; they can be sold in times of need. Ownership of one of any of these items added a further score of 1 to the household wealth index. Ownership of personal assets is significantly correlated with the housing score (Pearson correlation coefficient = 0.348, $P < 0.0001$), so those who have superior housing tend to have more personal assets.

[2] It will be appreciated that the term 'rich' here is being used, as by Polly Hill in Hausaland, with reference to local standards of wealth. In Mng'aru this means that absolute differences are small.

The Lorenz curve of the wealth index, divided by the number of adults in the household is shown in Fig. 7.3. The Gini coefficient is 0.404. Per adult wealth defined in this way is more equally distributed than individual ownership of trees.

How is this kind of wealth accumulated? One contrast with tree ownership is that while the latter increases with age, housing and personal assets are more extensive for younger household heads. There indeed appears to be no necessary relationship between ownership of tree crops and household wealth, especially assets. In the top 5 per cent of the cashew and coconut ownership distributions, only one person out of six in each case had more than one of the items included as assets. Old, tree-rich men do not buy personal assets.

Table 7.4 shows wealth and its component elements, and cashew ownership for households. In most cases only one person in the house (i.e. the male head) will own trees. While tree ownership clearly increase from an average of sixteen trees for household heads aged 30 and less to over eighty-five for those aged 70 or more, the household wealth index falls from 6.64 to 5. It is clear from looking at the component parts of the wealth indicator that this pattern is related to assets rather than housing. For household heads aged above 50 there is a sharp fall off in the number of assets owned, just as tree ownership rises substantially. The negative relationship between the age of the household head and asset ownership persists even when the number of adults in the household is controlled for. This age effect may reflect a generational shift, with younger men attaching greater importance to the acquisition of bicycles, clocks, and radios.

If age has no clear relationship with the housing indicator, previous migration to Dar es Salaam does. In particular, migrants are much more likely to have invested money in tin roofing (Table 7.5).

There is also a relationship between education and ownership of assets; there are more assets in the households of educated heads (Table 7.6).

Again, the factors here are co-variant; a multivariant test of significance shows that only migration remains important for the housing score.

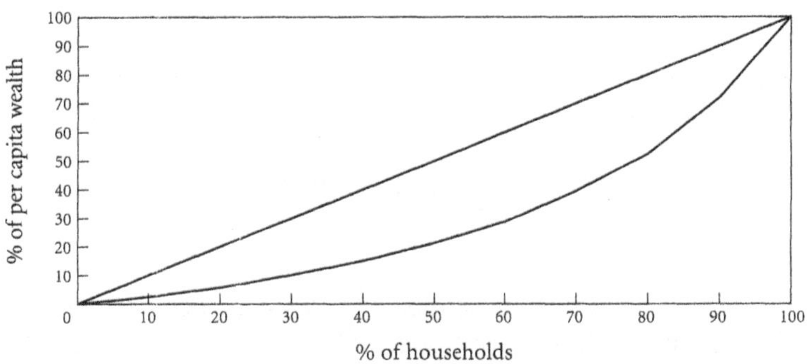

Fig. 7.3 *Distribution of per capita wealth*

Table 7.4. *Cashew and wealth ownership, by age of household head*

Age of household head	Mean cashews owned	Mean wealth index	Mean housing score	Mean no. of assets	*N*
<30	16.4	6.64	4.71	1.92	14
30–50	29.1	6.27	4.38	1.90	40
50–70	64.1	5.84	4.55	1.29	38
>70	86.2	5.00	4.39	0.61	28

Source: Household survey, Mng'aru, 1985.

Table 7.5. *Previous migration and roofing source (men aged 16 and over)*

Previous migration to Dar es Salaam	Roofing		
	Nyasi	Makuti	Mabati
No	39 (31.4)	74 (59.7)	11 (8.9)
Yes	2 (9.1)	13 (59.1)	7 (31.8)
Chi-square 11.308, 2 d.f., $P < 0.005$			

Source: Household survey, Mng'aru, 1985.

Table 7.6. *Education of household head and asset ownership*

Education	Mean no. of assets	*N*
None	0.73	48
Colonial primary	1.54	22
Adult education	1.71	31
Modern primary	2.47	19

Source: Household survey, Mng'aru, 1985.

Education and marital status are significant for asset ownership, but only marital status survives as a factor in overall wealth.

One further factor which might be expected to have a strong bearing on household wealth would be the sex of the household head. Female-headed households are often found to be overrepresented amongst the poorest. However, there is little difference between male- and female-headed households in Mng'aru in terms of housing, while the mean number of assets owned is 1.5 and 1.0 respectively.

Accumulation and Economic Activity

The final, and most important aspect of accumulation in Mng'aru concerns how wealth, in terms of both trees and assets, is related to economic activity. This is addressed here in two different ways. First, there is the question of whether wealthy men or households participate more in other high-return agricultural or extractive activities. If they do so, such activities may be an important part of accumulation strategies. Second, are there important differences between poor and wealthy households in time allocation? This issue has implications not only for understanding accumulation paths, but also for the analysis of relationships between demographic factors and time-use which is carried out in Chapter 9.

Relating tree ownership with the propensity of the household to grow rice, a high-value crop, reveals no significant association. On the other hand, there is a positive relationship, significant at the 5 per cent level, between rice growing and the household wealth index. Eighty-seven per cent of those households with a wealth score of 7 of more grow rice, while only 53 per cent of those with a wealth score of 4 or less do so (Table 7.7).

However, it is also true that household composition changes with wealth, and aspects of this, especially the number of women, are shown below to be important factors in whether a household grows rice or not. Therefore, what is required is a measure of wealth which is independent of household labour supply, i.e. wealth per adult. This measure is not significantly related to rice-growing. Wealth does not, therefore, have an independent effect on a household's ability to grow rice; but wealthier men marry more wives, or wealthy households attract more female relatives, which in turn means that these

Table 7.7. *Rice-growing, household composition, and wealth*

Wealth index	Percentage growing rice	No. of men	No. of women	Size	*N*
<4	53	1.0	1.1	4.25	32
5	77	0.9	1.1	4.65	31
6–7	73	1.1	1.2	4.52	33
8+	88	1.3	1.7	6.00	24

Source: Household survey, Mng'aru, 1985.

households are more likely to grow rice. These points are taken up again in Chapter 8.

When it comes to non-farming activities, the participation of members of households by the wealth of households and their heads depends very much on the definition of wealth. This again shows the distinct accumulation strategies for cashews, coconuts, housing, and personal assets. Looking at cashew ownership first, the only clear patterns are that those who have no cashews tend to be more involved in off-season crafts (such as carpentry and brewing) and extractive activities (such as charcoal preparation). This could reflect labour clashes, since these activities are pursued in the months following the rice harvest (i.e. August onwards), and cashews are harvested in September to October. However, for some crafts, especially carpentry, this pattern may also reflect the finding above that cashews are accumulated more by old men, while carpentry is done largely by younger men. Brewing, equally, is a woman's activity, and women own few cashews. No activity stands out as positively implicated in cashew accumulation except farming. Those with no cashews are indeed those who are most diversified in their non-farming activities.

For coconuts, the patterns of craft and charcoal production also apply, but there is a clearer positive cluster of activities associated with coconut ownership. There include trading, fishing, and wage labour. However, the numbers involved are still relatively small, so that these activities will only be potentially important as accumulation strategies for a few.

In the accumulation of household wealth, including housing, by contrast, poorer households do more trading, but this is reversed taking the number of adults into account. Other activities make little difference, except wage labour. Again, the number of people who gave this as a secondary occupation is small, but they are more often found in households with more wealth, but less wealth per adult. This suggests that they are found in large households, an issue which is returned to in Chapter 9.

Finally, in examining the relationship between wealth per adult and the allocation of time by household members, the difference between men and

Table 7.8. *Wealth per adult and men's labour allocation* (minutes)

Activity	Wealth per adult		
	<1.5	1.5–2.5	>2.5
Productive tasks	202	275	302
Domestic tasks	16	31	39
Personal needs	172	246	205
N	20	32	40

Sources: Household survey, Mng'aru, 1985 and time-use surveys, Mng'aru, 1986.

women once again appears. Wealth per adult has no significant impact on women's time-use, but it does on men's (Table 7.8). Men in wealthier households spend more time in productive activities than in those in poorer households. This finding differs from that of Gillian Hart in Java. There, she found that poorer men worked longer hours, but had less income (Hart 1980: 191). The positive association here between wealth and income-earning labour time suggests a greater reliance on household (male) labour. There is also, of course, a reliance on women's domestic and agricultural labour, which does not go down with wealth.

8 Households and Life Cycles in Mng'aru: Norms and Patterns

In order to understand how demographic events and the evolution of households may affect people's patterns of work, we need accounts of the life cycle of the household and of individual lifecourses. The first step is to grasp what a household in Rufiji is, and how it relates to the organization of labour, consumption, accumulation, and residence, and to the development of families. There are two ways of looking at this. The first is in terms of norms, or social ideals of what a proper household is like, or what a normal life cycle is. The second is the varied pattern of actual life cycles and household structures.

Compared to the simple model of a family household in Chayanov, or even in Binswanger and McIntire, the picture of household organization and structure in Mng'aru which emerges is considerably more complicated. First, households are not the only groups in which labour is organized, and in particular, sub-household groups of men and boys, or women and girls, are important for cooperation in gender-specific tasks. This makes the sex composition of a household as important as, if not more than, its age composition.

A scond feature of households in Mng'aru is that a number of factors make the life cycle of households much more complex than the Chayanovian model (or indeed that which is the norm in Mng'aru itself). Some of these factors are to do with the pattern of reproduction which arises out the demographic history described in Part I, namely sterility and marital instability. Others are to do with various ways in which households are extended to include non-nuclear kin, and with polygyny.

Households in Rufiji

At the most elementary level, households in Rufiji are apparently easily recognizable. There are no large compounds, such as those in West Africa containing many married couples and other relatives (e.g. Hill 1974). Rather, the 'typical' household consists of a married couple with children, living in a single house, farming a number of fields between them.

On closer examination, however, households in Rufiji, like households elsewhere in many parts of the world, are difficult to pin down (Yanagisako 1979).

At this point it is more useful to use the neutral term 'domestic group'. Part of the reason for this difficulty is that domestic groups on the coast of Tanzania differ in membership and structure according to their functions. However, it is also because, while there is considerable variation in the composition and workings of domestic groups within a community, and even from day to day, there are also notions, or norms about how domestic groups operate which give a much more permanent and well-functioning picture. Both norms and real variation are part of the reality of 'households', and so both must be considered. In this section I am largely concerned with the ideal forms of households; that is, how people represented households to me.

In term of residence, ideally each adult or adult couple lives separately, either in a house (*nyumba*) or a hut (*kibanda*). However, even when this is the case, and often it is not, because people's social affiliations are typically geographically widespread, there is a lot of coming and going. As Prins observed: 'A distinctive trait of the *nyumba* is its lack of consistency in personnel' (Prins 1967: 79).[1]

What may be called a (commensal) household exists at the level of eating together from a main kitchen. This unit also perhaps corresponds most closely to what the Tanzanian state identifies in Rufiji as an administrative household, the *kaya*. Since men will consider it demeaning to cook where there is a woman present, the ideal commensal household always involves a woman, or at least a teenage girl.

By contrast, as outlined in Chapter 6,[2] production groups are both larger and smaller than commensal households or residential groups. Both communal labour parties, and subgroups of mothers and children, co-wives, fathers and sons, or simply individual house members, constitute labour groups. These groups, distinct from residential and commensal households, have a curious notional existence. They are readily recognized; as one old woman put it to me, '*Kila mtu analo shamba lake*'—each person has their own field. However, the idea of semi- or even fully autonomous production groupings within a household clashes with the notion of the control a man has over his family.

[1] As an example of this lack of consistency, the following is the history of the household in which I lived between December 1985 and September 1986. Before I moved in, the household consisted of a man in his forties, A, his wife, son from a previous marriage, aged about 15, and a daughter aged about 5. In December his wife left him and went to live with relatives in Zanzibar. The daughter went to stay with her grandmother in the village. At this point I moved in.

January: a cousin of A's arrives, with her teenage daughter. They start preparing to farm rice in the valley.

February: A's son argues with his father, and leaves for relatives in Mkongo. A's daughter comes back to the house.

April: The visiting cousin moves to a *dungu* in the rice fields. Her daughter, together with A's daughter, lives half there and half in the village. A's son returns for a short time, and then leaves again.

Late May/June: A's cousin and her daughter harvest rice and return to the village. They then go off to a village on the road to Dar es Salaam to visit her husband.

Throughout this period, A would go to Dar es Salaam for a few days every month, where he acted as a rent collector for someone. The cousin's husband would also come at weekends from the other village, where he was a teacher.

[2] See also Caplan's discussion of Mafia Island (1981: 102–3).

In this sense, 'intra-household' conflicts, for instance over the rice that women grow, is as much to do with a clash of notions to do with family authority on the one hand, and the autonomy of production within a household on the other, rather than straightforward competition for economic gain.

Finally, property—trees, houses, personal items including beds, cooking implements, clothes, etc.—is owned by individuals, rather than a conjugal or familial estate or by a larger grouping, such as *ukoo*. Women ideally receive a number of items on marriage which constitutes her household wealth, including beds, cooking pots, clothes, etc. This can be added to in subsequent years. Women in theory inherit according to *sheria* (Islamic law), but as the actual distribution of wealth shows, women often do not gain personal control over their inheritance. However, the principle of individual ownership of personal wealth still applies.

It is thus by no means straightforward to identify 'the (peasant) household' as an economic and residential unit, and to describe its developmental cycle, even at the level of notions. This is perhaps best illustrated in a linguistic point. Despite its appearance in countless reports and books on Tanzania, there is no word in Kiswahili which conveys the various levels of meaning of 'household' in English. As noted, one official term is *kaya*, but this is rarely in everyday use in Rufiji. On the other hand, there are the words used to denote houses (*nyumba*) and huts (*kibanda*), but these are not really households either, although they may sometimes be commensal households. What is revealing is how people in Rufiji themselves denote what we would call a household—by the Kiswahili preposition *kwa*—which in this context means 'place of', together with the name of the person who is the head of the household. Thus 'old man Lisapwike's household' is denoted *kwa mzee Lisapwike*. At a certain level, this demonstrates the dominance of the concept of family over that of household. It is clear that this factor was at work when I attempted to get a sample of households for the time budget interviews. Each ten-cell leader was asked to select seven households at random for inclusion in the sample. Although there are a fair number of single-person households in the village, and half of these are headed by women, most of those selected by the ten-cell leader had married couples in them, and none was female-headed. This is partly because the *kwa* formulation is not used so easily to refer to such households, since they are not 'proper' households. *Kwa* literally means 'at the place of', but it is clear that, for the ten-cell leaders of Mng'aru, a place (household) cannot belong to a single woman in the same sense that it can to a man.

Life Cycles in Rufiji

Family is central to the identity, if not the various functions, of a notional 'household' in Rufiji. It is thus useful to have an idea of how the notional (or 'proper') and actual life courses of individual men and women fit together with the life cycle of domestic groups.[3]

[3] For definitions of the life cycle and life course, see Harris (1987).

We start with the experience of children, and young people up to marriage. Children in general are encouraged to be independent from as early an age as possible—starting to farm, fish, and trade from their very early teens or before.[4] Another general feature of the early life course is a process of status transformation through a series of rites and other events, culminating in marriage. However, while the process applies equally to boys and girls, the particular series of transformative experiences are very different in each case.

The central rites in ritual and ceremonial terms are related to sexual maturity, and are called *unyago* for both sexes.[5] While the female *unyago* is of enormous significance in status terms, the boy's *unyago* is less so. It occurs at circumcision, which marks a state of cleanliness and preparedness for marriage and adulthood. Names given at birth are abandoned for new ones.

The next significant life-course event for young men is a period in which they move out of their parents' house and live in a hut or *kibanda*, usually near by the main house. They usually continue to eat with their parents, thus still constituting part of a 'household'. This move is based on respecting the privacy of both boys (now, unlike girls, regarded as social adults) and parents; it was explained to me as allowing the boy to come and go as he pleased, often late at night, without disturbing others in the house.[6]

At this stage young men have an ambivalent relationship with the parental house in terms of labour. While still having responsibilities in familial labour contributions, they also form the main demographic group within the wage-labour force, and sometimes their own expenditures clash with the demands of their duties, leading to disagreements. This leads to the paradox that young men, as a group, are perceived as those with visibly the most leisure time, while they are simultaneously the main source of wage labour, both local and migratory. The paradox is partly explained by young men's relation to the land. Notionally, unmarried men do not farm substantial acreages on their own account (and in fact few do). This is partly because married men receive priority in *ukoo* allocations of recently cleared land. Unmarried men could in theory cultivate any bush land, but since such work involves a substantial minimum fixed input of labour, and since the youth has no family to support, the small plots, which are all that is needed, are not worth farming. Wage work on a larger plot worked by someone else may thus offer returns at a rate between the marginal product of labour at very small and at larger scales. It also provides flexibility across time, so that the young man is not 'tied' to the land across the entire season or even on specific days. This enables him to be available for his filial duties, as well as providing flexibility in leisure. This flexibility and mobility—thoroughly incorporated into the masculine concept of a 'youth' (*kijana*, *mhuni*)—also formed the primary economic and cultural basis for sex and age specificity in migration to Dar es Salaam.[7]

[4] See Caplan (1982: 36–7) and Swantz (1970) for comparative accounts.

[5] For full descriptions and symbolic interpretations of the coastal rites, see Swantz (1970: 185–200) and Caplan (1976).

[6] See also Caplan (1981: 103).

[7] *Mhuni* strictly translates as a vagabond or wastrel, and was in the past used to refer to 'free' women. Its use has become increasingly specific to young men.

Such freedoms, and the status of social adult inferred by the *kibanda* arrangement, are the antithesis of unmarried female experience (e.g. Caplan 1981: 103). Common to coastal and non-coastal societies in eastern Tanzania is the manner in which the transition from the status of girls to that of adult married women is a long process or series of events (Cross-Upcott 1956: 198; Swantz 1970: 185; Caplan 1976: 26). However, central to this process, in the case of girls, is the ceremony connected with puberty (*unyago*, *ngoma kutoa mwali*), which includes teachings about relationships between men and women, and between relatives, and about sex, menstruation, and birth. If a suitor has been found, this ceremony is often combined with a wedding, completing the transformation. It is important to note that puberty and marriage are of much more weight in conferring status than is childbearing;[8] according to older women in Mng'aru, childlessness does not incur a lack of respect, it is seen rather as bad fortune. Thus it is *fecundity* which is important rather than *fertility*.

Previously, an integral part of this phase of female rites was a period of seclusion. During this time, the girl, called a *mwali*, would have to stay in one room of the house, observing a number of avoidance taboos and performing only light work.[9] It is clear, however, that there has been a universal and steady decline in the significance of this institution, especially with the advent of universal primary education.[10] Periods of seclusion from menarche to marriage of five years or more were common, but now the norm is nearer a few weeks, often just before the wedding. Equally, although the practice is still said to be universal, the conditions of seclusion are no longer so strictly observed.

Data from interviews with women in Ikwiriri showed proportions secluded as *mwalis* falling from around 0.95 for those born before 1950 to around 0.3 for those who reached puberty after the introduction of universal primary education.[11] Declining prevalence of seclusion has gone hand in hand with shorter seclusion for those who do become *mwalis*, falling from a reported average of twenty-seven months for the oldest age group to under ten months for the youngest.

The *mwali* institution has many symbolic interpretations, but an obvious social one is the control of women's reproductive capacity.[12] Older men thus associate the breakdown of seclusion, and the presence of unmarried teenage women in public space, with premarital sex and 'illegitimate' births. In practice, the *kibanda* arrangement for young men makes premarital affairs easy to conduct.

'Illegitimacy' in this meaning is present, but unusual, incurring parents' anger, but not their rejection. Premarital pregnancy is in fact far-reaching in

[8] See also Tanner (1962: 78) and Caplan (1976: 26).

[9] For a full account see Swantz (1970).

[10] See also Caplan (1981: 103) and Swantz (1985).

[11] See Swantz (1985) for vivid accounts of how parents in Ikwiriri resisted education for girls precisely because it clashed with the *mwali* institution.

[12] The control of female sexuality in this context is more complex, and present more centrally in the *unyago* ceremonies themselves rather than in seclusion.

life-course terms in its implications for marriage. By far the most important female marriage in Rufiji is the first one, and thus also the one in which parents are likely to have the most influence. In the balance between the parents' and the child's decisions about partners, with all the implications for the conjugal relationship, a premarital pregnancy can force the issue, even if one partner is not in fact so keen.

It is generally maintained that parental arrangement of marriages has declined, both over time, and in relation to groups of outsiders, such as 'Arab' traders. Indeed, as early as 1937, colonial administrators in Utete were writing that arranged marriages were 'extinct'; marriages were now made by the contracting parties without reference to parents (RH 1937). However, most first marriages still involve a large degree of parental and kin participation, not least because of the orchestration of payments and gifts to the bride and to bride's kin. It is possible that what the perception relates to is a decline in the practice of child marriage of brides. This is described at length by Cross-Upcott (1956: 198–209), and effectively involved the betrothal of a child and suitor, with extended labour service, and eventual marriage upon puberty.[13] Certainly, child marriage meant greater parental power in decisions, although the ease of early divorce in these cases is described as giving the girl an effective veto (ibid. 246). Child marriage also kept female age at first intercourse low, and was attributed by one observer to be a factor in a very high mortality rate for first born children.[14] Age at first marriage has probably risen significantly since the 1930s (see Chapters 1 to 5).

Upon first marriage, unless the groom was a much older man, or already with other wives, the 'normal' pattern is for the couple to go and live initially with the father of the groom. This period facilitated the absorption of the wife into the life of the husband's kin, and the preparation of a house and farm.

In the 'ideal' life cycle, the domestic group then goes through a period of expansion as the couple have children who grow to maturity. Actual life cycles, as we shall see, diverge from this norm according to different experiences of infecundity, polygyny, the arrival of other kin, divorce and separation, and mortality.

The fostering of children is a common phenomenon in Africa, both East and West (Goody 1982; Nelson 1987; Page 1989). However, 'fostering' often implies a fairly permanent adoption of a child. While this does occur, so that children may spend ten years with a grandparent, or with a childless relative, the movement of children also includes shorter stays, ranging right down to a few days. Long-term fostering to childless couples or grandparents is a well-developed form of 'smoothing out' demographic variation between houses, and as such it is backed by considerable moral sanction. It is considered *moyo mbaya*, i.e. meanness, without heart, to refuse either to let children go to such a couple, or for the couple to refuse to take the children. Thus, Pat Caplan

[13] See also Swantz (1985: 33–4).

[14] Interview with Fr Robin Lamburn, Kindwitwi, 17.7.86.

argues that children's movements can be treated partly in terms of the claims of kin who have rights in them (Caplan 1984: 36).[15]

It is not clear that fostering institutions can be interpreted as fulfilling primarily economic strategies. There are, in principle, a wide range of motivations at work. As mentioned below, divorce may lead to difficulties for mothers, and temporary fostering by a child's grandmother or parents sibling is often a solution. Remarriage, however, can equally lead to problems, as men are often unwilling to maintain another man's children (Caplan 1984: 36–7) so that temporary arrangements can become permanent. Most significantly, it has been observed that children make their own decisions about where they want to live: they often decide where and when they would like to go and stay with a relative, and when they want to return. It is worth noting that much fostering goes on between closely related kin, especially the siblings of parents and grandparents. The corollary of this is that grandparents and parents' siblings play an important role in socialization and ritual.

For the adult married man and woman, interdependent life courses can develop in a number of ways. Specifically, couples can stay together, or separate; marriages can end in widowhood, or divorce. Marital instability has a number of consequences.[16] First, and most importantly, it demonstrates the ambivalent standing of women within the kin and marriage system. Rufiji's kinship is generally patrilineal, the cognatic systems of the coast have a patrilineal 'bias', and marriage in both cases is virilocal. On the other hand, divorce is relatively easy—as much because it has become accepted, as because of interpretation of *sharia*.[17] Landberg thus sees divorce as 'counterbalancing' patrilineal bias, since it means that the possibility of return to (female) natal kin exists.

On divorce, women generally, although not automatically, return to their natal village. This move is of importance because it eases conditions of economic survival for women who, in their husband's village, would have few resources with which to support themselves and their children. Many divorced women receive no financial assistance from the children's father, partly because this is one of the principal reasons for women obtaining divorces. In these circumstances, divorcees return to their natal villages because (i) they are more likely to own property (houses, trees) there, obtained through inheritance, and (ii) they are more likely to be able to find a supporting household to attach themselves to. The help of kin, especially female kin, with childcare and access to land, is seen by Landberg as central to the support systems for divorced women (1986: 116–28).

Divorced women in such situations may live in a *kibanda* adjacent to a relative's house, or build their own house. Such women face a particular burden of responsibilities, especially if, as noted, divorce arose from a husband's fiscal negligence. Indeed, one word used to describe divorce or separation in

[15] See also Tanner (1962).

[16] See Ch. 5 above for the history of marital instability on the Tanzanian coast.

[17] But see Caplan (1982: 83).

Kiswahili is *tumeasiana*—'we have abandoned our responsibilities towards each other'. Divorced women are thus often under pressure to fill both male and female parental roles, and they particularly need to earn cash. In Mng'aru, as elsewhere, this was done through brewing. Nine women in the village were known as brewers, or as agents selling beer, *ulaka*, and *gongo*. Of these, three were divorced, another three had husbands who were absent for long periods, and all were older women, having reached a stage in the life course where their eldest child had attained adulthood.

The origins of divorce should not, however, be understood here in purely economic terms. In a society where extramarital affairs are common for both men and women, but not condoned, marital instability is perhaps bound to be high. In this context, the great mobility of people, with women often returning seasonally to their natal villages to farm rice, and with the men going to Dar es Salaam for long periods, a high rate of divorce is associated by people themselves in Rufiji with conjugal separation and resulting extramarital affairs.

Whether married, single, divorced, or widowed, childless or not, for all surviving men and women, the life course ends in old age. Although illness can have a significant effect on productivity at any point during a lifetime, the old are the most likely to be infirm. However, even in such cases, the fundamental principle in relations between old and young is maintaining the independence of the former, as far as possible (Caplan 1981: 103–4). Old people continue to cultivate for as long as they can; they continue to live separately. Older widowed women often live in a *kibanda* adjacent to a son's or daughter's house. While elderly widowed men or infirm women will eat together with the main household, able-bodied women will continue to cook for themselves.

What is notable is the importance of rendering services—domestic and agricultural—to the elderly in this phase, rather than direct monetary support. It is relatively common for children above the age of 5 to go and live with grandparents, where they can perform the small tasks in and around the house that would otherwise become increasingly irksome for an elderly person.

The Case of the Missing Life Cycle

Chayanov's analysis of the peasant household evoked the notion of a single coherent life cycle, static, or changing only very slowly through historical time. However, there is considerable variation in the meaning, the extent, and the timing of these events described above across people and households. Examination of this variation shows that the notion of 'the life cycle' is somewhat of a chimera, dissolving into a series of divergent paths.

The aim in this section is to look at the patterns of (residential) households, relate this to the cycles of household formation and fission, and to see how these in turn generate demographic characteristics, such as age and sex composition. Some of these processes are also related to household wealth. This will help us to assess Chayanov's analysis of the role of life cycle in determining activity patterns through the dependency ratio, Binswanger *et al.*'s ideas about wealth and household size, and the role of life cycle in variations in sex ratios, and hence in the ability to cope with sexual divisions of labour.

Very little can be said, on the basis of the available data, about how the life cycle of residential groups in Mng'aru has actually changed. Survey data was gathered on current house structures only, and it is not possible to reconstruct past households accurately. Given this, there are two possible ways of proceeding. The first it to abandon all discussion of life-cycle factors, except for variation in residential groups *within* cohorts, based, say, on the age of the senior house member. The second is to start from an assumption that the current distribution of household types observed represents a more or less constant developmental cycle, and then adjust this view by making qualitative assessments on the basis of whatever material is available. Here we take the second course, and where possible address variation between cohorts as a subsidiary issue.

The starting point is some sort of characterization of the household life cycle. Categorizing life-cycle stages has become more complex since Glick's (1947) pioneering work in the 1940s and 1950s, as the restriction of the concept to nuclear families with stable marriages has given way to accommodate divorce, three-generational households, and one-parent households (Höhn 1987). In Rufiji matters are complicated further by the existence of joint households (i.e. with married brothers or sisters), households where other 'non-nuclear' relatives are also present, and polygyny.

An idea of this complexity can be got by taking the simple measure of the age of the most senior household member, and looking at the variation in household characteristics by life-cycle 'stage'. Table 8.1 shows the means and standard deviations of the number of children aged 6 years and under, for each life-cycle stage.

While the different stages are distinct in the number of young children present in the household, the standard deviations show the considerable variation within each stage. The period showing the least variation in the presence

Table 8.1. *Variation in number of children by age of household head*

Age	Mean	S.D.	Percentage with children	N
<30	1.2	1.28	63	16
31–40	1.8	1.57	81	16
41–50	1.7	1.11	79	29
51–60	0.7	0.91	44	18
61–70	0.3	0.56	28	25
>70	0.3	0.70	19	16

Source: Household survey, Mng'aru, 1985.

Table 8.2. *Marital status of household heads by age of household head*

Age	Single	Currently married	Divorced or separated	Widowed
<30	6	8	2	0
31–50	1	41	3	0
51–70	0	30	10	3
>70	0	11	2	3

Source: Household survey, Mng'aru, 1985.

Table 8.3. *Sex of household head by age of household head*

Age of household head	Male		Female	
	N	%	N	%
<30	13	81	3	19
31–50	39	87	6	13
51–70	35	81	8	19
>70	13	81	3	19

Source: Household survey, Mang'uru, 1985.

of young children is in the early mid-cycle, with household heads aged 30–50. These households also have the most children. It is thus clear that the distribution of young children is heavily concentrated in the early mid-life-cycle stage.

The effects of marital instability and extension also give rise to a range of different kinds of household being found at each life-cycle stage. A comparison of the marital status of household heads at different ages shows an interesting pattern (Table 8.2). Most household heads are married at every life-cycle stage. However, except for the 31–50-year age group, the percentage who are not currently married is never less than 20 per cent, and is 50 per cent for the youngest group.

A considerable number of households at each stage are headed by women (Table 8.3). The proportion of female-headed households is remarkably constant, at about 18–19 per cent, dipping only in the mid-life cycle.

There is also variation in the number and sex of active adults in households at each stage. Given the organization and gender division of labour described in Chapter 6, this showed important implications for economic activity. Table 8.4 shows a distribution of household types for each life-cycle stage. Type 1 households have one woman and no men aged over 16. Type 2 households have one man and no women. Type 3 households have one man and one woman, while type 4 comprises households with more than one of either sex.

No single household type contains more than 60 per cent of households in any one stage, and although multiple-adult households predominate, single-adult households form 25–30 per cent of the total in all stages except the 31–50 age group.

A final aspect of variation within life-cycle stages concerns household extension. Extension here means the inclusion of any household members who are not part of the nuclear family of the household head. Table 8.5 gives the percentage of nuclear and extended households, and the mean number of nuclear and extended members, for each life-cycle stage.

Table 8.5 shows that a third of households in each stage, rising to one-half for older household heads, contain non-nuclear members, while the majority do not. The average presence of non-nuclear members is small relative to the nuclear membership, but does not show a clear life-cycle pattern except in the last stage.

Table 8.4. *Variation in household structure by age of household head*

Age of household head	Household type			
	1	2	3	4
<30	1	3	6	6
31–50	2	2	15	26
51–70	6	6	12	16
>70	2	2	1	7

Note: Seven households having only adults recorded as economically inactive are excluded.

Source: Household survey, Mng'aru, 1985.

Table 8.5. *Variation in household extension by age of household head*

Age of household head	Nuclear			Extended		
	N	%	Mean no.	N	%	Mean no.
<30	11	69	3.4	5	31	0.5
31–50	30	67	5.3	15	33	0.6
51–70	30	70	3.5	13	30	0.6
>70	8	50	3.1	8	50	1.0

Source: Household survey, Mng'aru, 1985.

Table 8.6. *Distribution of households by type: Char Gopalpur and Mng'aru (%)*

Type of household	Char Gopalpur	Mng'aru
Subnuclear: single person(s)	10	23
Nuclear: married couple/trio and unmarried children	56	44
Supplemented nuclear: nuclear plus other single persons	19	26
Joint: two or more married couples	15	7

Source: Household survey, Mng'aru, 1985, and Cain (1978)

The household life cycle in Mng'aru thus turns out to be remarkably difficult to pin down in reality. In most life-cycle stages, especially for the oldest household heads, there is a considerable amount of difference between households and between household heads. The exception is really the mid-cycle stage, where heads are aged between 30 and 50. For this group we find that most household heads are married; more are men; the households have more members, and particularly more children. The implication of this pattern is that while households in Mng'aru form and develop in their early stages in a fairly distinctive manner, life-cycle patterns diverge rapidly after that.

One consequence of such a diverse life-cycle pattern is that the observed pattern of household types in Mng'aru at any one time is very varied. A useful comparison can be made with Bangladesh, where the central importance of the patriarch makes a single-household life cycle much clearer. In Mead Cain's study of 343 households in Char Gopalpur (Cain 1978), the distribution of household types in more concentrated than in Mng'aru (Table 8.6). In particular, the nuclear household is more common. By comparison, what Cain calls the supplemented nuclear household, and sub-nuclear (single-adult) households are more frequently found in Mng'aru, while joint households are relatively rare.

Life Cycle and Dependency Ratios

The contrast with Bangladesh is relevant for another reason. The fortunes of households there are strongly tied to the vicissitudes of the life cycle, and especially the presence of surviving sons, for three reasons (Cain 1978). First, the fact that household assets, such as land, can more easily be retained by men than by women. Secondly, the rigid sexual division of labour; and thirdly the relatively isolated nature of households, with little inter-household assistance.

As we have seen in Chapter 6, the nature of economic institutions in Rufiji mean that these factors are far less pronounced, enabling a wider range of households, especially single-adult and female-headed households, to persist. If the life cycle matters, therefore, it is more likely to matter in the Chayanovian sense, of the balance of workers and consumers at each stage. However, the diversity of life-cycle patterns implies that the simple relationship between life cycle and dependency ratios hypothesized by Chayanov will not be found in Mng'aru.

Before trying to identify patterns of dependency, we need to consider its definition. Since Chayanov's (1966) pioneering work, this has often been approached by constructing consumer and worker 'equivalents', and basing some measure on them, usually difference or ratio. Unfortunately there are problems with the rationale underlying this approach. For 'consumers', sliding scales are often based on nutritional models. However, there is an element of spurious preciseness here: such crude models are of dubious meaning, and are inevitably somewhat arbitrary. For constructing 'workers', a similar problem exists, since to avoid circularity, existing labour data cannot be used (Donham 1981: 523). For these reasons, there is little to be lost in using any reasonable arbitrary method of defining dependency. Here, since my primary interest is in the demographic aspect of dependency, i.e. age structures, I simply use the ratio of children aged 6 and under, plus adults unable to work, to active adults aged over 16 in the household, or the difference between them.

In Chayanov's original model, as the peasant family household went through the life cycle, the number of consumers relative to workers gradually rose to a peak, until children matured and began contributing to the workforce, so that the consumer–worker ratio fell again.

In Mng'aru, the matter is somewhat more complex. Figure 8.1 shows box plots of the spread of the difference between 'workers' and 'consumers' for each life-cycle stage. First of all, it shows that the median dependency difference does not rise and fall with the life cycle in the way posited by Chayanov, but rather, is constant. By contrast, the variation in dependency ratios *within* life-

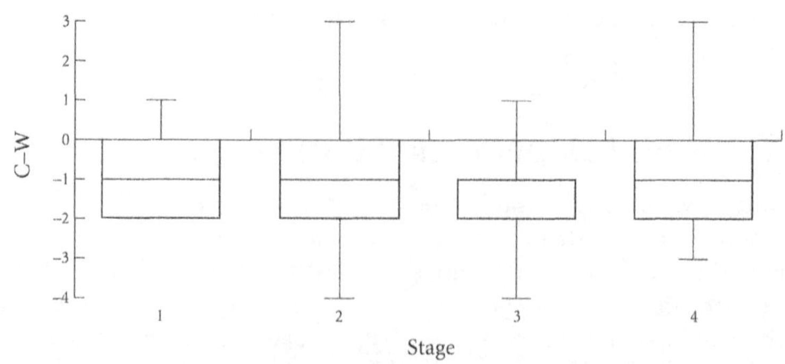

Fig. 8.1 *C–W differences by life-cycle stage*

cycle stages is large. This means that the association drawn by Chayanov between life cycle, dependency ratios or differences, and economic activity and mobility cannot be applied here. Dependency ratios may indeed be important for economic activity and mobility patterns, as indeed may other measures of age and sex structure, but there is no simple age-based life cycle that underlies differences in that structure.

Determinants of Household Structure

This leaves us with the question of what other factors influence household composition. Answers can be given at two levels. First, one can look at the immediate demographic processes which complicate the basic life cycle and cause variation in sex and age composition. Second, one can attempt to relate these variations in life-cycle patterns to underlying factors, such as that of wealth, suggested by Binswanger and others.

Infertility and marital instability

We have seen that two pervasive features of household composition in Mng'aru are (i) considerable variation in the number of children at each life-cycle stage, and hence in dependency ratios, and (ii) a relatively high proportion of households headed by single, divorced, separated, or widowed men and women. These features are in large part the result of two important aspects of the demography of Mng'aru (and indeed Rufiji generally): sterility and marital instability. The historical development of these phenomena has been described in Chapter 2.

An idea of the incidence of sterility can be gained from Table 8.7, which shows the incidence of primary and secondary sterility, for married women, by age group and by year of first marriage.[18] For comparison, of women aged 45–9 in the Coast Region in 1978, 11.9 had had no live births, and 21.7 had had 1–2.

There appears to have been a decline in the incidence of both primary and secondary sterility, perhaps especially in the latter. Testing for a decline in primary sterility only across year of marriage, and only for marriages contracted up to 1979, gives a positive result significant at the 5 per cent level (chi-squared = 13.043, 3 d.f., p = 0.011).

What does this pattern imply for the pattern of births and therefore the distribution of surviving children between women? Table 8.8 shows that the distribution is bimodal: while just under 40 per cent of women aged 35 and over gave birth to two or fewer children, just under 40 per cent gave birth to five or more. Mortality levels out the distribution of surviving children somewhat, reducing the upper tail. Nevertheless, there remains wide variation in the number of surviving children per woman.

The second factor is marital instability. A cross-section of current marital status is not very revealing on the question of change over time, since people

[18] Year of marriage here was calculated indirectly using current age and age at first marriage.

Table 8.7. *Primary and secondary sterility (married women, percentages)*

Group	No. of children			N
	0	1	>1	
Age group				
30–4	7.1	3.6	89.3	28
35–9	15.4	3.8	80.8	26
40–4	6.7	13.3	80.0	30
45–9	15.0	20.0	65.0	20
>50	25.0	15.4	59.6	52
Year of marriage				
1930–9	12.5	0.0	87.5	8
1940–9	39.3	17.9	42.8	28
1950–9	11.4	20.0	68.6	35
1960–9	13.3	15.0	71.7	60
1970–9	11.1	9.3	79.6	54

Source: Birth and marriage history survey, Mng'aru, 1986.

Table 8.8. *Parity and surviving children for women aged 35 and over, Mng'aru*

No. of children	Children ever born		Surviving children	
	%	Cum. %	%	Cum. %
0	13.7	13.7	17.8	17.8
1	11.0	24.7	12.3	30.1
2	12.3	37.0	11.0	41.1
3	4.1	41.1	4.1	45.2
4	8.2	49.3	11.0	56.2
5	15.1	64.4	15.1	71.2
6–7	22.0	86.4	22.0	93.2
>8	13.6	100.0	6.9	100.0
N	73		73	

Source: Birth and marriage history survey, Mng'aru, 1986.

can move in and out of the states of divorce and widow(er)hood, especially the former. Perhaps more useful is the average number of marriages per person. This is given for all women and for ever-married women only, by age group, in Table 8.9.

Table 8.9. *Mean number of marriages per woman*

Age group	All women	N	Ever-married women	N
25–9	0.8	29	1.1	22
30–4	1.4	30	1.5	29
35–9	1.8	27	1.8	27
40–4	1.7	31	1.7	31
45–49	2.0	21	2.0	21
>50	2.4	61	2.5	59
All	1.6	199	1.8	189

Source: Birth and marriage history surveys, Mng'aru and Ikwiriri, 1986.

Table 8.10. *Percentage distribution of women by number of marriages, Ikwiriri and Mng'aru*

No. of marriages					
0	1	2	3–5	>5	N
1.4	44.3	21.4	30.0	2.8	140

Sources: Birth and marriage history surveys, Mng'aru and Ikwiriri, 1986.

Concentrating on the age groups over 30 years, where never-married women constitute a negligible group, it is clear that age is associated with a higher average number of marriages. Whether this is due to a real decline in marriage instability, or incomplete cohorts, it is impossible to say. However, with a sample mean of 1.8 marriages per ever-married woman, and with over two marriages per woman over the age of 45, at least one divorce is the norm.

However, how many women actually follow the norm? Looking at variation within rather than between cohorts, table 8.10 shows the percentage distribution of women aged 35 and over, by number of marriages. As can be seen in the table, there is substantial variation in experience between women who are reaching the end of their reproductive years. Almost one-third have been married at least three times, while 46 per cent have been married no more than once.

As might be expected, marital instability is related to sterility; women who have been married often tend to have fewer children (Table 8.11). This association may be for a number of reasons: because of long periods between marriages; because a larger number of sexual partners increases the probability of contracting gonorrhoea; or, more likely, infecundity in women leads their husbands to divorce them and remarry.

Table 8.11. *Number of children ever born by number of marriages, women aged 35+, Mng'aru*

Children ever born	No. of marriages		
	1	2	3+
0–2	10 (26)	5 (36)	22 (73)
3–5	10 (26)	5 (36)	5 (17)
6+	19 (49)	4 (29)	3 (10)
Total	39 (100)	14 (100)	30 (100)

Source: Birth and marriage history survey, Mng'aru, 1986.

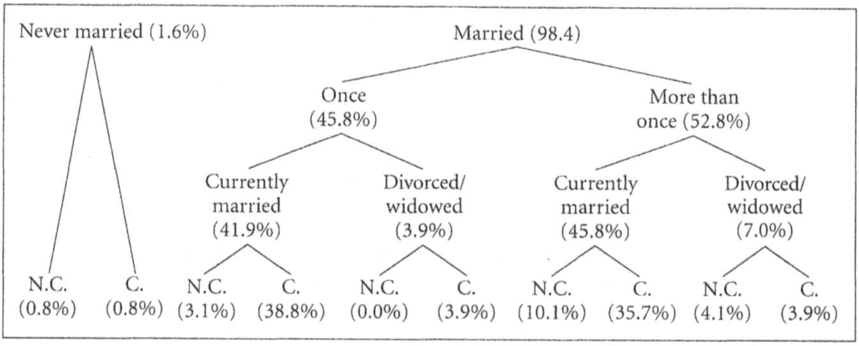

Fig. 8.2 *Life-course paths for women aged 35 and over*

Combining marital experience with fertility experience gives us a picture of life-course paths for individual women. Figure 8.2 shows the percentage distribution of women aged 35 and over in Mng'aru and Ikwiriri by their life-course path. By following the arrows, more detailed breakdowns are given: by whether the woman has ever been married, number of times married, current marital status, and whether or not she has borne children. The figure shows that, along these particular lines, life-course experience by age 35 is fairly concentrated. Almost three-quarters of these women are in two categories: those currently married, having borne children, and married once or more than once. Variation thus appears to be generally of *degree* rather than *type*: most women have marriages, and most women have children; the difference lies in how many.

Current marital status also of course affects the sex composition of the household: almost all households with both active adult men and women in them have household heads who are currently married. Households with 'unbalanced' sex ratios have predominantly unmarried heads.

These demographic patterns are important inasmuch as they help us to make sense of some of the diversity in life-cycle experience. However, birth is not the only way of building a household, and marital instability for individuals does not preclude the strategic use of marriage to affect household size and composition. The next two sections examine the importance of polygyny and extension as more conscious methods of managing household structure, and therefore their association with wealth.

Polygyny, household composition, and wealth

The first, and most obvious strategy for a wealthy man to enlarge his household and the labour potentially available to him is polygyny. Relatively few men in Mng'aru are polygynously married, and most of them are older. Of the twelve polygynously married men (household heads) in the sample, seven were over 50, and eleven were over 40.

Polygyny is associated with the wealth of the husband, measured in terms of housing and assets. It is less clearly associated with the ownership of tree crops. However, polygyny is in turn clearly linked to the ability to farm more: households headed by polygynously married men farm almost a third more land overall, and more than double the acreage of rice, of those headed by monogynously married men.

The strong relationship between wealth and polygyny can be seen in Table 8.12. Three-quarters of the polygynously married household heads are in the richest category.

What relationship does polygyny have with household structure? Not surprisingly, the outstanding feature is more women. Households headed by monogamously married men have on average 1.34 economically active women (N = 69), while those with polygynous heads have 2.41 (N = 12). The latter also have more teenagers and young children, but the differences are smaller.

Thus polygyny explains part of an important element of household

Table 8.12. *Wealth and polygyny*

Wealth indicator	Unmarried		Currently married: monogamous		Currently married: polygamous	
	N	%	N	%	N	%
<4	14	44	17	53	1	3
4–5	11	36	19	61	1	3
5–6	7	32	14	63	1	5
>6	7	20	19	54	9	35

Source: Household survey, Mng'aru, 1985.

composition—sex ratio. However, polygynous households are relatively rare, and polygyny has no clear relationship with the dependency ratio.

Household extension and wealth

Another way in which household composition can be directly influenced by decision is through new members being absorbed, often relatives. Such household extension is, as we have seen, more common in the very late stages of the life cycle.

What kind of people are thus absorbed, and what kind of households do they end up in? Here, an extended household has been defined as one containing non-nuclear family members of the household head. It thus includes stem households.

First, we may note that, as with polygyny, household extension is associated with total household wealth, as measured by housing and personal asset indicators (Table 8.13).

However, household extension is widespread at all levels of wealth. Overall, forty-one households, or about one-third of all households in the village, had extended members.

Does extension serve the function of 'balancing' dependency or sex ratios? In order to answer this question, we need to examine both the household as it would have been without additional relatives, and who those relatives are themselves. Taking dependency structures first (Table 8.14), there is no clear relationship between a high or low dependency ratio in the 'nuclear' component of the household, and a balancing ratio in the extended component. Especially for housholds whose nuclear components has more workers than consumers, household extension seems to reinforce rather than offset this. Conversely, households with more consumers than workers (or a balance) in their nuclear components, do not generally get help from their extended elements.

Similar results hold for sex ratios (Table 8.15). Nuclear and extended components are distinguished by whether they have both men and women aged 16 or over in them, either men or women, or no active adults at all, i.e. only adults who are not in the labour force.

Table 8.13. *Wealth and household extension*

Wealth group	Nuclear			Extended		
	N	%	Mean no.	N	%	Mean no.
<4	24	75	3.88	8	25	0.38
4–5	24	77	4.29	7	23	0.35
5–6	13	59	3.82	9	41	0.73
>6	18	51	4.42	17	49	1.09

Source: Household survey, Mng'aru, 1985.

Table 8.14. *Net consumer–worker differences for extended households: nuclear and extended components*

Nuclear component	Extended component		
	+ve	0	−ve
+ve	1	2	3
0	6	0	1
−ve	9	10	9

Source: Household survey, Mng'aru, 1985.

Table 8.15. *Sex composition of extended households: nuclear and extended components*

Nuclear component	Extended component			
	Neither	Female	Male	Both
Neither	1	2	0	0
Female	2	4	0	0
Male	3	2	1	0
Both	9	8	6	3

Source: Household survey, Mng'aru, 1985.

Most nuclear components contain both men and women, but the few that have not tend to have female extended components. Of nuclear units which have either a man or a woman, there is no particular tendency to have an extended component which balances the sex ratio. In the majority of cases, they have extended components with only the infirm or elderly, or with the same sex as themselves. These results are slightly different if we allow for girls and boys aged 7–15, in that there tends to be more balancing. However, the majority of cases (68 per cent) still have both male and female members in the nuclear components.

What Tables 8.14 and 8.15 reveal is that household extension is mostly of two types. First, there is the absorption of an elderly, infirm relative, often a parent. Secondly, there is the taking in of divorced or separated women with their children. Those not in the labour force, and women with children, make up about three-quarters of the cases of household extension in Mng'aru.

The relationship with wealth therefore needs to be interpreted carefully; clearly richer households can afford to take on relatives in need. However, they also benefit from them. An elderly parent may not be able to farm, but is often able to help look after children or do domestic tasks. A divorced woman may not only grow rice, but will also generally help in domestic work.

Conclusions

The main conclusion to be drawn from this examination of household forms and life-cycle processes in Mng'aru is that models of household labour supply based on a single coherent life cycle do not capture a complex and fluid reality. Rather than a single life cycle over which households follow, there are a multiplicity of patterns in Mng'aru. For most households, there is a mid-life-cycle stage where: the household is headed by a monogamously married man; there is a high dependency ratio because there are young children and few older ones; and there is a balanced sex ratio. After this, there are broadly three main routes. In the first, the household head marries again to form a polygynous household, which has a lot of young children, teenagers, and more women than men. The second and third possibilities arise out of separation and divorce. These lead to single-headed households which typically have very unbalanced sex ratios. The multiplicity of life-cycle paths means that at any one time there are a great many distinct household types in Mng'aru. With a unitary life cycle, we will observe different types at any one time because housholds pass through different stages. Here we are looking at a pattern which arises out of different stages *and* distinct paths.[19]

Household size, age, and sex composition are influenced by factors other than a simple life-cycle variable (such as age of head). Maritial instability, fertility differences, polygyny, and household extension all influence the structure of a household. It is to the implications of these for work patterns that we now turn.

[19] As Caplan notes, the fluidity of form depends partly on the flexibility of temporary housing—the *kibanda*—for three types of people: teenage boys, divorcees, and old people (Caplan 1981: 102–3). What is striking is the perseverance of these forms in the face of villagization and campaigns for *Nyumba Bora* (better housing) in the 1970s.

9 Household Demography and Patterns of Work

Seif Ali Tangu lived near the centre of Mng'aru, in a small house on a field which sloped down towards a valley to the west of the village. In 1986 he had nine children, and in August his wife delivered another. There were seven children aged under 12 years. The eldest boy, a 20-year-old youth, was living in Dar es Salaam. Seif Tangu and his wife were responsible for feeding and clothing all the other children between the two of them. This they could barely manage, and coping with their dependency burden left little time for trying any strategies of accumulation. The family were living in a house built out of palm thatch, which began to fall down in the long *masika* rains. Tangu had plans to build a more permanent house, but these had been indefinitely postponed.

Early on in our acquaintance, I asked him why he grew so much cassava, which is a low-value crop in both monetary and nutritional terms. 'And if I did not, what would my children eat?' he replied. His answer is clearly partly to do with the many risks involved in growing a high-value crop, selling it, and then buying food. However, it also reflected the fact that his farming decisions, and the amount of work he did, were consciously influenced by the family he and his wife had produced. Seif Tangu is an extreme example, someone whose large dependent family dominated his activities. With no adult children living in the village, and with his wife pregnant, 1986 was a hard year, since Tangu himself had to do most of the cultivation. However, all the households in Mng'aru, with a handful of exceptions, face the same fundamental problem: how to balance the needs of household members with their labour resources, without a ready wage-labour force to make up imbalances.[1]

This chapter is thus about the relationship between current household structures and work patterns in Mng'aru. It attempts to go beyond particular, often dramatic, cases, to provide a quantification of which factors are important for most households in Mng'aru. It is important to state at the outset that one of the main findings is that household composition explains only part of the story. Patterns of wealth explain even less, however. Networks of cooperation and mutual help in both domestic work and rice-growing, the data

[1] His example also shows that the problem is rooted in time. Later on, if his children are successful, and remain loyal to him, Tangu will have a large group of offspring to rely upon. His problems today will be balanced by rewards later on, although, as I have argued above, I do not believe that this is *why* Tangu has so many children.

suggest, may explain more. But these lie largely beyond the scope of this study, and can be described only in outline.

However, the data are of value in developing the way in which household composition and work patterns can be analysed. In particular, they show the limitations of the standard approaches described in the Introduction to Part II. The models outlined there hypothesize a number of relationships between general household characteristics, such as size and consumer/worker ratios, and patterns of activity. In the first section of this chapter, these are assessed and tested in the case of Mng'aru. It quickly emerges that these aggregate characteristics hide more important and interesting aspects of household structure, which are addressed in the following sections. The labour-allocation patterns of men and women are not only very different, but they also respond differently to variations in household structure. A particular focus is brought to bear on two key activities of women—household maintenance and rice cultivation.

The findings suggest that it is important to understand divisions of labour in Mng'aru not simply in terms of sex and age-specific tasks within a 'household farm', but also in terms of the relationships of each person to the others in the household, and to others outside. In this sense, in spite of land abundance and the relative smallness of the labour market, simple demographic models of the household are of limited relevance here. They are thus conditional not only on interhousehold labour and relations in the market for land, but also on non-market relations between groups and individuals within and between households.[2]

The demographic measures used in this chapter were introduced in Chapter 8. Some of the measures of work and activity were used in Chapter 6. The three main kinds of economic measure are: (i) diversity of activities, e.g. farming, fishing, charcoal preparation, etc.; (ii) time spent in production, domestic work, and in personal reproduction, including leisure; and (iii) whether people grow rice, and how much is grown. Rice was chosen as part of the focus on women, since it is largely a 'woman's crop'. Indeed it is, as described in Part I, of central importance to women's incomes. It was in general, in 1985–6, a valuable crop.

Household Structure and Activity Patterns

We have seen in Chapters 6 and 7 that Rufiji has some of the characteristics found in models of peasant economy from Chayanov, Binswanger, and others. In particular, labour supply comes largely from the household, and the supply of land is reasonably flexible. Under these conditions, we would expect household size and composition to have a significant influence on patterns of activ-

[2] This point has, of course, been made on many occasions. See Guyer (1981) for an excellent exposition. On the absence of gender relations from the Chayanovian model in African contexts see Hunt (1979) and Low (1986). Unfortunately, gender is not analysed in the more recent Binswanger *et al.* work; they limit their analysis of intrahousehold relations to intragenerational cooperation and conflict.

ity. At the same time, we saw in Chapter 8 that household size and composition do not follow, as they do in Chayanov's simple model, from a 'household life cycle'. This is because rather than a single coherent life cycle, in Rufiji there are many diverging paths.

Household size and economic activity

The first aspect of household structure to be examined is also the simplest—overall size. The Binswanger model predicts that size makes no differences to cultivation per worker, but this is qualified by the need to control for differences in age and sex. It also implies that activity per worker declines for very large households because of supervision costs. This is supported by Shapiro's work on Zairean households (Shapiro 1990). By contrast, Low (1986), building on the work done by Nag *et al.* on child labour contributions, and on Chayanov's notion of 'complex cooperation', argues that larger households are more efficient, and may take part in a wider range of productive activities. Toulmin found this to be the case in Mali (1992).

Do working members of large households work more than those in smaller households? Are they involved in a wider range of activities? Are they more involved in high-return activities? Table 9.1 shows the relative diversity of activities undertaken in households of different sizes in Mng'aru. All adult household members were asked about their activities. Virtually everyone in Mng'aru defined themselves as *mkulima*, or farmer. However, more diversity emerged when other, dry-season activities were asked about. The majority still had no other major activities, but some did. The table thus shows, for each activity and for two measures of household size, i.e. number of people and number of adults, the percentage of households in which that activity was named.

It is clear that larger households are more diversified. In a higher proportion of larger houses, people are fishing, making charcoal, and doing wage work. Most of the difference is between the smallest households and the rest.

Turning to rice cultivation, Table 9.2 shows that small households as a whole participate in rice-growing less than larger ones. However, as emerges below, this hides a contrast between male- and female-headed households. Note also that, at the household level, there is no difference in rice-growing activities between households with three to five members and those with six or more.

The most direct assessment of the relationship between household size and worker efficiency and activity is given in Table 9.3, which shows average time spent per day on productive work and household maintenance by each active adult, by household size.

Only a small number of adults in the time-use sample were in the smallest households. The larger samples for the two larger household size groups show little difference in per adult work hours in domestic tasks. Adults in the largest households spend somewhat less time in productive work than in medium-sized households.

Table 9.1. *Household size and household participation in secondary activities*

Activity	Household size					
	1–2		3–5		6+	
	N	%	N	%	N	%
Farming	17	59	39	93	49	100
Fishing	3	10	3	7	13	27
Trading	1	3	3	7	1	2
Charcoal/ extractive	1	3	4	10	5	10
Wage labour	2	7	4	10	7	14
Crafts	1	3	4	10	4	8
Cooperative activities	0	0	1	2	4	8
N	29		42		49	
Activity	No. of adults in household					
	1		2		3+	
	N	%	N	%	N	%
Farming	10	33	35	88	50	100
Fishing	2	7	5	13	12	24
Trading	1	3	3	8	1	2
Charcoal/ extractive	0	0	6	15	4	8
Wage labour	1	3	2	5	10	20
Crafts	2	7	5	13	2	4
Cooperative activities	0	0	0	0	5	10
N	30		40		50	

Source: Household survey, Mng'aru, 1985.

Finally, both the Chayanovian and the Binswanger models imply that the amount of land that a household farms will be positively related to the size of its labour force, i.e. its number of workers. Here, the evidence generally supports this hypothesis, although the relationship is not monotonic (Table 9.4).

Larger households in Mng'aru are therefore systematically different from smaller ones. Larger households contain within them people doing a wider range of activities, and they are more likely to have someone growing rice in them. They also cultivate more land altogether, as hypothesized by Chayanov, Binswanger, and others, although the area cultivated per head decreases with

Table 9.2. *Household size and rice-growing*

	Percentage of households growing rice	Mean acreage of rice	N
Household size			
1–2	52	1.4	29
3–5	79	1.9	42
6+	78	1.9	49
No. of adults			
1	57	1.6	30
2	73	1.6	40
3+	80	2.0	50

Source: Household survey, Mng'aru, 1985.

Table 9.3. *Per adult labour allocation and household size*

Activity	Household size		
	1–2	3–5	6+
Minutes			
Productive tasks	209	257	213
Domestic tasks	88	210	204
Per cent			
Productive tasks	29	36	30
Domestic tasks	12	29	29
N	10	63	144

Source: Household survey, Mng'aru, 1985 and time-use survey, Mng'aru, 1986.

Table 9.4. *Mean acreage of land farmed, by number of adults (aged > 16)*

No. of adults	Acres	N
1	1.9	20
2	4.1	38
3	3.9	40
4+	5.4	22

Source: Household survey, Mng'aru, 1985.

household labour force, which contradicts Binswanger and McIntire's basic hypothesis. Equally, adults on average spend less time on productive work in larger households, so any gains that there might be from 'complex cooperation' do not show up in time-use terms.

It is clear, however, that knowing about household size in fact tells us rather little. For instance, we know from Chapter 6 that there is a strong sexual division of labour in Rufiji, so that a household with two women is likely to be different from one with two men. Equally, a household with six members could consist of six active adults or, rather like Seif Tangu's household, it could have one or two adults looking after young children or elderly relatives. We therefore need to look at the age and sex composition of households and at dependency ratios.

Chayanov's rule and some exceptions

The central question here is whether or not Chayanov's rule applies, i.e. that workers in households with a higher number of dependents, relative to workers, have to work harder. Table 9.5 shows that there is no simple relationship for productive work, taking households as a whole.

The first group consists of households with many more workers than consumers, and the third group mostly of those with a balance, or more consumers than workers. Time per adult spent in productive work is somewhat higher for those in households with a high c–w measure and those with a low measure, and slightly less for those in the middle range. By contrast, there is a clear relationship between dependency burden and the amount and percentage of per adult time devoted to household maintenance.

Why does Chayanov's rule not apply? The answer is straightforward: figures for time-use averaged out over the household conceal sharp contrasts between men and women (Tables 9.6 and 9.7).

Table 9.5. *Per adult labour allocation and consumer–worker differences*

Activity	Consumers–workers		
	<–1	–1	0+
Minutes			
Productive tasks	225	212	244
Domestic tasks	186	212	215
Per cent			
Productive tasks	31	31	35
Domestic tasks	25	31	31
N	101	55	55

Sources: Household survey, Mng'aru, 1985 and time-use surveys, Mng'aru, 1986.

Table 9.6. *Male labour allocation and consumer–worker differences*

Activity	Consumer–workers		
	<–1	–1	>–1
Minutes			
Productive tasks	242	296	326
Domestic tasks	29	36	33
Per cent			
Productive tasks	34	42	48
Domestic tasks	4	5	5
N	50	19	22

Sources: Household survey, Mng'aru, 1985, and time-use surveys, Mng'aru, 1986.

Table 9.7. *Female labour allocation and consumer–worker differences*

Activity	Consumers–workers		
	<–1	–1	>–1
Minutes			
Productive tasks	208	167	190
Domestic tasks	339	304	336
Per cent			
Productive tasks	28	25	26
Domestic tasks	45	45	46
N	51	36	33

Sources: Household survey, Mng'aru, 1985, and time-use surveys, Mng'aru, 1986.

The pattern for men shows a strong Chayanovian effect—as the c–w difference rises, so does men's labour-time input. Their low level of domestic work remains the same. For women, the overall labour input drops slightly as the c–w difference increases, while their domestic labour is largely unaffected, remaining high. Regardless of the consumer–worker difference, women in all groups spent on average almost half of their day in domestic work.

Household age or dependency composition thus does matter, but more for men than for women. This implies that sex composition matters as well as, or indeed more than age composition. However, it is also clear that further analysis of the effects of demographic structure on labour allocation must treat men and women separately.

Sex composition and economic activity

Participation in a wide range of activities in Rufiji is sharply differentiated by sex (see Chapter 6). Looking at the size of households regardless of their composition may miss important differences in the range of activities covered by households. This is seen in Table 9.8, which for various activities gives the percentage of households taking part in those activities, by household type. Type F consists of households with one adult woman, type M, one adult man. Type FM households have one man and one woman, while type FFMM households have more than one man, woman or both.

Note first that, unlike as in Smith and Sender's study of the Usambaras (1990), female-headed households[3] are not involved at all in wage labour. It is the largest and most varied households which contain people doing the most wage labour, although these are still a minority. This represents both a strong sexual division of labour, the limited labour market, and alternative sources of cash income for female-headed households in Mug'aru. They are generally still amongst the poorest households, but they can obtain small cash incomes from brewing and selling beer, marketing cooked foods, and above all from selling rice.

Households with a single adult man but no women have a more diverse range of activities than those with just women, but in turn are not as diversified as the larger households which contain at least one man and woman.

The contrast between men and women also emerges in the case of participation in the high-value crop of rice, especially since, as emerged in the discussion of historical change, rice has become a 'woman's crop'. Table 9.9 shows the relationship between rice-growing and the sex composition of households. The number of men in a household is negatively associated with a household's likelihood of rice participation. By contrast, there is a strong positive association between the number of women in a household and participation in rice. Where there are more women in a household, those growing rice also grow more.

The relationships between household characteristics and activities at the household level tell us a certain amount. Larger households (which we saw in Chapter 8 tend to be the households of wealthier men) have an advantage over smaller households. But beyond this, the factor of overwhelming importance is gender. Much of the attributable variation in household time allocation and rice-growing patterns is due to the sex composition of households. However, men and women not only have different patterns of work, they also have different responses to household demography, as we saw with consumer–worker differences. It is therefore not enough to regard the sexual division of labour

[3] Note that, although type-F households are generally female-headed, some female-headed households are included in category FM, because they have an adult son or other male relative in them.

Table 9.8. *Household type and household participation in secondary activities*

Activity	Household type							
	F		M		FM		FFMM	
	N	%	N	%	N	%	N	%
Farming	10	91	8	62	32	94	53	96
Fishing	0	0	2	15	5	15	12	22
Trading	3	27	1	8	3	9	1	2
Charcoal/ extractive	0	0	0	0	6	18	4	7
Wage labour	0	0	1	8	1	3	11	20
Crafts	1	9	1	8	4	12	3	6
Cooperative activities	0	0	0	0	0	0	5	9
N	11		13		34		55	

Note: seven households recorded as having no active adults were exclused.

Source: Household survey, Mng'aru, 1985.

Table 9.9. *Household sex composition and rice cultivation*

Sex	Percentage of households growing rice	Mean acreage of rice	N
No. of men			
0	77	1.9	26
1	71	1.8	66
2+	68	1.8	28
No. of women			
0	50	1.8	22
1	72	1.5	61
2+	84	2.3	37

Source: Household survey, Mng'aru, 1985.

simply as consisting of static distinct male and female contributions to a common farming or productive unit. As we saw in Chapter 6, for Mng'aru this is unjustified in any case. Men and women have different kinds of relationships to the household, and to others within (and outside) the household. To trace some of these relationships, it is necessary to look, not at the allocation of labour and rice-cultivation decisions at the household level, but rather at individual level patterns.

'A Woman's Work is Never Done'

Women's work patterns have already been identified in the analysis in this chapter and Chapter 6. However, an overall sexual division of labour acts as a set of limits for the amount and type of work that women do. Within those limits there may be considerable variation in the problems and opportunities facing individual women in different circumstances. Two sets of factors are considered here: individual characteristics and household characteristics.[4]

Individual characteristics

Here we consider the significance of the individual characteristics of women—their age and marital status. Their possible importance lies in their relationship to variations in the social and economic roles of women in Rufiji. First, age is an important indicator of experience, and since rain-fed rice is a long-established crop in Mng'aru, older women may know more about it than younger women. Age is also an indicator of social status, and young women may be more likely to carry out certain tasks than older women. Secondly, getting married is an important step for women in Rufiji society. It often marks entry into independent cultivation on one's own account, with access to land made much easier. As wives, women also become part of kin groupings which cooperate in certain stages of rice-harvesting and processing. Equally, divorcing, or becoming a widow may also have an impact on rice cultivation. Finally, monogynous and polygynous marriage place women in different situations, and senior and junior wives also play different roles. All of these factors may influence rice-growing and domestic labour patterns.

Taking age first, older women grow rice more, and grow slightly larger acreages, although the difference is not significant for the latter (Table 9.10).

Secondly, marital status affects the likelihood of a woman growing rice, although again the acreages grown by women of different marital status vary little (Table 9.11). Note the particular role played here by marital status, in a situation where land for rice-growing is readily available in absolute terms. The biggest contrast is of course between unmarried women and the rest. However, amongst the other categories, divorced and separated women stand apart from married and widowed women in their lower propensity to grow rice. This may be due to the small sample or to co-variant features of household composition. However, it may also be due to the direct relationship

[4] Many different characteristics were explored, but some were quite co-variant. Thus, for example, unmarried women tend to be young, while divorced and widowed women tend to be older, so that marital status and age are co-variant. To avoid confusing the effects of two distinct factors, the multivariate general linear models (GLM) procedure in the statistical package SAS was used to generate tests of significance. Only those factors significant at the 10% level were selected for further analysis in the text.

Table 9.10. *Women's age and rice-growing*

Age	Percentage growing rice	Mean acreage of rice	N
16–29	34	1.3	50
30–44	67	1.5	51
45–59	69	1.5	29
60+	74	1.6	23

Source: Household survey, Mng'aru, 1985.

Table 9.11. *Women's marital status and rice-growing*

Marital status	Percentage growing rice	Mean acreage of rice	N
Single	5	(3.0)	20
Married	68	1.5	107
Div./sep.	50	1.4	18
Widowed	63	1.3	8

Note: The figure in parentheses is for one observation only.
Source: Household survey, Mng'aru, 1985.

between marital status, rice land, and harvesting. Rice land is in principle available to all, but areas of rice land in the valley are associated with particular *ukoo* groups. Women's rice-farming is organized through their husband's kin. Thus if they are married, or widowed, their status within the *ukoo*, and their claims to land, remain more legitimate. Divorced and separated women, by contrast, are in an anomalous position. Not only are they now no longer part of their husband's *ukoo*, but they are also often marginal within the households and kinship hierarchy of their natal home. This means less assistance with getting cleared land, and perhaps most importantly it excludes them from the mutual working groups of women who harvest, thresh, and winnow rice collectively. These groups are based on extrahousehold relationship to a patrilineage through birth or marriage. The women in these groups are almost always married, as opposed to divorced or widowed women.

A woman's marital status also strongly affects her allocation of time. This remains true even when taking age into account. In the time-use sample there were few widowed or divorced women, so the comparison is largely between married and single women.

Time allocation and rice-growing are thus both clearly related to marital status: married women, because of their status, have easier access to the

Table 9.12. *Women's labour allocation and marital status* (minutes)

Activity	Currently married	Not married
Productive tasks	204	135
Personal needs	131	196
N	95	26

Sources: Household survey, Mng'aru, 1985, and time-use surveys, Mng'aru, 1986.

productive resource of land, and therefore work longer hours in productive labour. They of course are also more likely to have more children. However, their status clearly involves different expectations and responsibilities to those of unmarried, divorced, or widowed women.

By contrast with marital status, age is not a significant factor in the determination of time-use for women.

Household characteristics

The individual characteristic of a woman can have a strong effect on her labour allocation, including the decision to grow rice. However, as argued above in Chapters 4 and 6, women act neither in a vacuum, nor simply as undifferentiated 'household members', but rather in particular relationships to other members of the household and others outside the household.

We saw above that the consumer–worker difference had little impact on the time-use patterns of women (as opposed to men.)[5] However, the absolute number of young children (6 years or less) in the household in which a woman is living (usually, but not always, her own children) does make a difference, for both productive time and domestic labour (Table 9.13)

Women with young children do less productive work and more domestic work. Those with two or more children aged 6 or less spend almost an hour longer per day on domestic labour.

Work by Theresa Ho (1979) on women's time-use patterns in the Philippines showed that teenage girls are an important substitute for their mother's time in domestic labour, allowing the latter to pursue market employment. This is similar to Nag *et al.*'s point about children freeing adults' time in large households. In Mng'aru, however, the pattern appears completely different (Table 9.14). Teenagers appear not to release productive time for the adult women in their households, but to lead to those women spending more time on domestic work, whether or not they have young children. While the numbers for those without young children are small, the result still holds for those with young children, where the sample size is larger.

[5] This was also true of a dependency ratio, giving the ratio of dependants to workers within households.

Table 9.13. *Number of young children and women's time-use* (minutes)

Activity	No. of young children		
	0	1	2+
Productive tasks	252	195	167
Domestic tasks	289	309	343
N	21	31	69

Sources: Birth and marriage history survey, Mng'aru, 1986, and time-use surveys, Mng'aru, 1986.

Table 9.14. *Women's time-use by presence of young children and presence of teenage girls (aged 12–18)* (minutes)

Activity	Without young children		With young children	
	No teenagers	Teenagers	No teenagers	Teenagers
Productive tasks	255	247	184	187
Domestic tasks	267	342	307	355
N	15	6	48	46

Sources: Birth and marriage history survey, Mng'aru, 1986, and time-use surveys, Mng'aru, 1986.

A more detailed look at the time-use categories shows where that increase lies (Table 9.15). Taking only those women with young children, the biggest switch is away from time spent on cooking and towards time spent directly with children. From these data, therefore, it appears that teenage girls release mothers' time which they use in childcare, rather than in farmwork.

What is the effect of young children, and hence the burden of domestic work, on women's rice-growing? Does having young children prevent women from growing rice? In fact, it makes little difference to the decision to grow rice, but does slightly affect the amount grown (Table 9.16).

Why do young children not have a stronger impact on the rice-cultivation patterns of women? First, because of its organization, whereby women can be resident in *dungu* in the fields, most of the processes of rice-growing are reasonably compatible with the care of an infant or toddler. Through the wet season, vegetables can be grown around the *dungu*, providing a food supply. Most importantly, there need not be long distances to walk from home to fields, especially where a relative or older child can bring necessary items from the village. Supporting evidence for this is that although women with

Table 9.15. *Amount of time spent in domestic work by adult women with young children and with and without teenage girls*

Domestic activity	No teenagers		Teenagers	
	Minutes	%	Minutes	%
Childcare	18	6	57	16
Cooking	140	45	133	37
Firewood collection	8	3	8	2
Food preparation	63	20	82	23
Water collection	63	20	56	16
Washing dishes/ sweeping	16	5	21	6
Total domestic work	308	100	357	100

Sources: Household survey, Mng'aru, 1985; birth and marriage history survey, Mng'aru, 1986; and time-use surveys, Mng'aru, 1986.

Table 9.16. *Women's rice-growing and young children in the household*

No. of children	Percentage of women growing rice	Acreage of rice grown	N
0	54	1.5	63
1	48	1.7	48
2+	53	1.3	59

Source: Household survey, Mng'aru, 1985.

young children do grow rice as often as those without, they farm smaller areas: acreage farmed rises steadily with the age of the youngest child in the household.

Secondly, the period of maximum incompatibility between childcare and rice cultivation is relatively brief for each child. Looking at levels of participation in rice-growing and the age of the youngest child in the household, the pattern shows a drop to about 40 per cent of women with children aged between 2 and 4 years, but nearer 60 per cent for women with infants and older toddlers (Fig. 9.1). The latter group can be left alone or with an older child, while the former can be carried. It is when children are too heavy to be carried, but not old enough to be independent, that they are a burden.

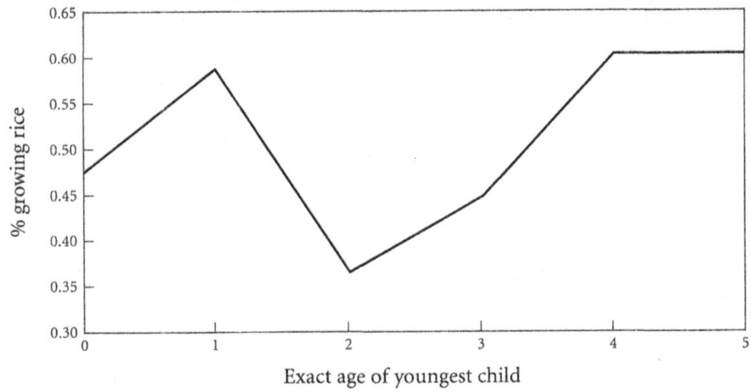

Fig. 9.1 *Women's rice-growing and children's ages*

Table 9.17. *Number of women in the household and women's time-use* (minutes)

Activity	No. of women		
	1	2	3+
Productive tasks	171	196	209
Domestic tasks	337	325	300
N	43	58	20

Sources: Household survey, Mng'aru, 1985, and time-use surveys, Mng'aru, 1986.

Thirdly, there are means of spreading the burden of childcare through help from relatives and older children, especially where the burden is seen to be heavy.

The overall demands of child-rearing in the community may be both rising over time and equalizing in incidence as sterility decreases. However, the pattern of time-use and participation in rice-growing outlined above shows that women will try to maintain their involvement in the latter, again demonstrating the value attached to claims to an independent cash income.

Apart from their marital status, and the number of young children in the household, the main factors affecting the time-use patterns of individual women are the absolute numbers (rather than the ratio) of men and women in the household (Tables 9.17–9.19). Where women are on their own in a household, they spend significantly more time on domestic-labour, and less on productive work. This effect is independent of the number of young children in the household, and provides evidence for cooperation between women in the

Table 9.18. *Women's rice-growing and number of women in household*

No. of women	Percentage growing rice	Acreage of rice grown	N
1	69	1.3	61
2	48	1.6	54
3+	42	1.7	31

Source: Household survey, Mng'aru, 1985.

Table 9.19. *Number of men in the household and women's time-use* (minutes)

Activity	No. of men		
	0	1	2+
Productive tasks	219	193	173
Domestic tasks	280	311	363
N	12	69	40

Sources: Household survey, Mng'aru, 1985, and time-use surveys, Mng'aru, 1986.

same household, spreading the load of domestic work, and freeing labout time to spend on cultivation.

A similar pattern can be seen in women's rice-growing (Table 9.18). For women who are the only woman in the household, 69 per cent grow rice, and these 69 per cent grow on average 1.3 acres. In households with more than one woman, the likelihood of any one woman growing rice drops sharply, suggesting that there is a division of activities, so that one woman concentrates on rice cultivation, while the other(s) do complementary tasks which help her. This is supported by the fact that women growing rice in such households grow larger acreages.

The impact of men on women's time is quite different from that of other women (Table 9.19). In quite a dramatic way, Table 9.19 shows that the presence and number of men in the household is associated with less productive work for women, and a considerable increase in the amount of domestic labour they perform. The impact of men on women's time-use is diametrically opposite to that of women.

Men's Allocation of Labour

The time allocation of men is also strongly affected by a few key variables. Generally, the most important of these are marital status and the number of other men in the household.

First, the contrast between married and unmarried men can be seen in Table 9.20. Married men spend almost twice as long, every day, on productive labour as unmarried men, and about an hour less on personal needs.

These differences reflect the key difference between the demands on the perceived responsibilities of married men on the one hand, and those of unmarried men on the other. Comparison with Table 9.12 above shows that marital status influences time allocation in a similar way for men and women.

The same is true of the main element of household composition significantly affecting men's time-use—the number of other men in the household (Table 9.21). Once again, the presence of other men means less productive work and more domestic work.

This result may reflect the fact additional men to the household head will often by young, unmarried men, or elderly men. Both of these types of men

Table 9.20. *Men's labour allocation and marital status* (minutes)

Activity	Currently married	Not married
Productive tasks	321	168
Personal needs	185	267
N	62	30

Sources: Household survey, Mng'aru, 1985, and time-use surveys, Mng'aru, 1986.

Table 9.21. *Number of other men in the household and men's time-use* (minutes)

Activity	No. of other men	
	0	1+
Productive tasks	322	233
Domestic tasks	8	48
N	39	53

Sources: Household survey, Mng'aru, 1985, and time-use surveys, Mng'aru, 1986.

are more likely to do more domestic work, and less fieldwork, than household heads.

The time that men spend on domestic labour is also significantly affected by the number of young children in the household. Men with one young child spend only nine minutes a day on average on domestic work, while those with three or more spend fifty-five minutes. Even this figure is far lower than that for women, however.

The most striking negative finding is that men's time allocation is not significantly related to the number of women in a household. The amount of time they devote to their productive activities is therefore largely independent of women.

Work and Domestic Organization

Aggregate household size, and even dependency ratios, tell us relatively little about work patterns in Mng'aru. Although larger households contain a membership more diversified in their activities, the allocation of labour time and participation in various activities is in fact dominated by the gender division of labour. At the simplest level this means, as is fairly obvious, that the sex composition of a household is a key determinant of the activity undertaken within that household. Indeed, sex composition appears to be rather more important than age composition.

However, the gender division of labour means more than this. For in Mng'aru, few activities are undertaken by whole households as such, but rather by individual men or women, or by sub- or extra-household groupings. What matters here is that men and women's use of time, and decisions to participate in different activities, respond to individual characteristics, and to the make up of the households in which they live, in quite distinct ways. They have different relationships with the other members of the household, and with others outside of the household.

These issues are particularly important for women when it comes to growing rice, because rice is a high-value crop, and is a major source of income for women over which they can legitimately claim control. One of the more important factors affecting the rice-growing activities of individual women is their marital status, which I have argued is in turn related to their access to land, and to networks of other married women based on kinship, during the process of harvesting and threshing.

Existing models of the household have difficulty dealing with such phenomena. The most general set of models considered here has been those developed by Binswanger and others. However, like most other models of the household, it assumes that the basic issue is how work is allocated amongst a household labour force. This approach is reflected in empirical applications, such as Shapiro (1990). But in the case of women's rice-farming in Mng'aru, the issue is not one of the allocation of labour between the members of a unified household, but rather of (i) explaining why, when groups are formed in the processing of rice, they are often not households, but rather extra-household kin-based groups; and, (ii) competing claims of family members over the product of cultivation undertaken by individuals (or a household subgroup).

Thus, models of the division of labour must be able to accommodate more than one domestic group, and explain the differences between them. Further, they must be able to distinguish between different kinds of cooperation and conflict (Sen 1985). This is most clearly seen in the second point raised above. Sometimes husbands or other male relatives cooperate in the labour process of growing rice, and claim part of the crop based on their contribution. However, conflict over the rights to rice proceeds between husbands and wives also arise when men claim rice not on the basis of any contribution, actual or perceived, but rather on the basis of a household or family relationship—being a husband or a brother. Cooperation and conflict is thus not one-dimensional.

Understanding conflict is particularly important in the case of Mng'aru, precisely because so many larger households splinter into smaller ones. Although there are clear advantages to living in larger households, divorce and separation are still very common, and there are relatively large numbers of single-headed households. Although life is typically more difficult for people living in those households, since they have inflexible labour resources, unbalanced by gender, it is nevertheless the case that they result from larger households which failed to cohere.

Conclusion

In this book I have tried to provide an analysis of reproduction which works on two levels. The first—the substantive content of the study—itself falls into two parts. One is an account of how social and economic change has influenced biological reproduction, especially fertility, in coastal Tanzania over the course of the twentieth century. The other is an investigation of how demographic factors shape economic constraints and actions at the individual and household level in one village.

But the intent is to provide not simply an analysis of a particular demographic history, or household labour organization in a particular village, but also a template for the understanding of reproduction more generally. This template is based on the premiss that biological reproduction, the reproduction of the labour force, and social reproduction are all interrelated, but not in functional or deterministic ways.

In each half of the book, a methodology is developed from this premiss. The analysis of fertility builds out from the demographic trends, through the proximate determinants, which then 'point' to specific social and economic institutions or arenas of behaviour as likely candidates for explaining fertility change.

In the case of coastal Tanzania, the application of this methodology produces evidence for stagnant and then rising fertility after 1950, based on a regime of early marriage, marital instability, and long birth intervals. Change was caused by a slowly rising age at first marriage, increasing divorce rates, and a shortening birth interval. The social and economic history of coastal Tanzania suggests that these proximate determinants—marriage and birth intervals—are rooted in political and spatial organization and a gendered economy. These in turn were transformed by Islam, villagization, and colonial economic transformation to produce conjugal conflict, marital instability, and new parameters for marriage formation.

But the key point about this methodological template is that, applied to another place and another time, the particular story will be different. Nor does such a methodology presuppose any particular social, economic, or cultural theory of fertility change. Indeed, the purpose of the approach is to identify the dimensions of demographic change, and work outwards from there, rather than choosing a theoretical frame and then fitting demographic change into it.

It is useful to consider in what ways such an approach differs from more conventional, functionalist accounts. First, it is by necessity historical, since it is impossible to understand what influences fertility without considering how it changes. Second, in seeking to discover what determines fertility, the approach leads towards explanations located not at the level of individual utility, but rather at the level of institutional or social structure and change.

Finally, it is important to locate the particular account here and the more general methodology, in relation to the study of 'demographic transition'. This study has looked at shifts in fertility within a 'natural fertility' population. This is not to say that there is no fertility control, but it is to say that there is an absence of conscious individual fertility control based on achieving a certain number of live births. The use of modern contraceptive methods in Rufiji District and coastal Tanzania more widely remains very low.[1] This is therefore not a book about demographic transition. However, if there had been a fall in fertility over the period, and a large rise in the use of contraception visible in the movement of proximate determinants, this would have formed a central part of the study. However, as before, the underlying explanation for this could not be assumed (to be for example, a rise in child costs, or a decline in the influence of African religion) but would have to be pursued in the historical and anthropological record.[2]

The second half of the book is also a study of how various levels of reproduction interact, but from a rather different perspective. It focuses on the relationship between biological reproduction and the formation of the labour force. Within peasant societies, this topic is the focus of a debate going back to the beginning of this century, with Lenin's and Chayanov's works on the Russian peasantry.

In the case of Rufiji, land availability means that household demography does play a major role in determining the labour supply. This is broadly Chayanov's position, but a crucial departure is in seeing household demography—and the labour force—as socially as well as biologically constructed. Polygyny and household extension through fostering and sheltering relatives play a major role. The other main point is that gender divisions of labour, socially determined, heavily influence the relationship between household composition on the one hand, and work patterns and diversity of activities on the other. Finally, at the level of individual women, their demographic experience and status—both marital and reproductive—does influence work, but this influence is mediated by who else is in the household, and by the woman's relationship with others outside the household.

There are various lessons to be drawn by comparing this approach with other accounts of peasant economies. One obvious one is that the reproduction of the labour force does not follow on immediately or determinately from biological reproduction. A second is that, very often, the relations involved in reproducing households—both biological and social—have been overlooked in the focus on the presence or absence of wage labour.

[1] Although even if it were higher this would not necessarily imply a sudden shift to parity-specific fertility control (Lockwood 1996).

[2] For exactly such a paradigmatic account, in a case where contraception use has risen without much change in fertility, see Bledsoe *et al.* (1994).

A great deal of emphasis in this book has been placed on the possibility and importance of separating out different levels of reproduction, and identifying non-deterministic or non-functionalist relationships between those levels. This concept of levels of reproduction is an abstraction. In reality, the conception, birth, and raising of a child to become a working, social adult, involves reproduction at all three levels, interweaving in a way which is inextricable in lived experience. However, the claim to analyse fertility change, or the role of household demography in economic life, must attempt some analytical separation if it is to move beyond either simple description, or a mechanical ascription.

References

1. Archival Sources

Two main sets of colonial archives were consulted. These were the annual reports from Rufiji District held at the Tanzania National Archives in Dar es Salaam, and the District Books for Rufiji held at Rhodes House Library, Oxford University.

(*a*) District Reports

These are referred to in the text by their accession numbers, prefaced by the latters TNA. All are annual reports for Rufiji District, except where indicated.

TNA 1733/1	1919–20 (Kilwa, Kisarawe, and Rufiji Districts)
TNA 1733/5	1921
TNA 1733/17/1/10	1924
TNA 1733/18:105	1925
TNA 61/3/VI/D	1931
TNA 61/3/IX/D	1934
TNA 61/3/XI/D	1936
TNA 61/3/XIII/D	1940 (monthly reports)
TNA 61/504/1/I	1946
TNA 61/504/1/III	1951

(*b*) Tanganyika Secretariat: Memoranda from the Principal Medical Officer

TNA J9 19153/I	1923–35
TNA J9 19153/II	1939–44

(*c*) District Books

These consist of observations and histories collected by colonial administrative staff. They are held at Rhodes House Library in Oxford on microfilm, reel MF 32, the originals being in Dar es Salaam. Some of the books are dated, while some of them are undated but divided into sections with short title. In the text the Books are referred to by the letters RH and either the date or the section title, whichever is appropriate.

2. Other Sources

Adegbola, O. (1977) 'New estimates of fertility and child mortality in Africa, south of the Sahara', *Population Studies* 31/3.

ALLEN, J. W. T. (1981) *Desturi wa Waswahili of Mtoro bin Mwinyi Bakari and other Swahili Persons*, Berkeley and Los Angeles: University of California Press.

ARENS, W. (1975) 'The Waswahili: the social history of an ethnic group', *Africa* 45/4.

Bank of Tanzania (n.d.) *Tanzania: Twenty Years of Independence*, Dar es Salaam.

BANTJE, HAN (1979) *The Rufiji Agricultural System: Impact of Rainfall, Floods and Settlement*, Research Paper 62, Bureau of Resource Assessment and Land Use Planning, University of Dar es Salaam, Dar es Salaam.

—— (1980) *Floods and Famines: A Study of Food Shortages in Rufiji District*, Research Paper 63, Bureau of Resource Assessment and Land Use Planning, University of Dar es Salaam.

—— (1987) 'Seasonality of births and birthweights in Tanzania', *Social Science and Medicine* 24/9.

—— (1988) 'Female stress and birth seasonality in Tanzania', *Journal of Biosocial Science* 20.

BARDHAN, P. (1989) *Economic Theory of Agrarian Institutions*. Oxford: Clarendon Press.

BARNUM, N. H., and SABOT, R. H. (1977) 'Education, employment probabilities and rural-urban migration in Tanzania', *Oxford Bulletin of Economics and Statistics* 39/2.

BEARDALL, W. (1881) 'Exploration of the Rufiji River under the orders of the Sultan of Zanzibar', *Proceedings of the Royal Geographical Society*, 3.

BECK, ANN (1977) 'Medicine and society in Tanganyika', *Transactions of the American Philosophical Society* 67/3.

BECKER, GARY (1960) 'An economic analysis of fertility', in A. Coale (ed.), *Demographic and Economic Change in Developed Countries*, Princeton: Princeton University Press.

BECKER, GARY (1981) *A Treatise on the Family*, Cambridge, Mass.: Harvard University Press.

BELSEY, MARK (1976) 'The epidemiology of infertility: a review with particular reference to sub-Saharan Africa', *Bulletin of the World Health Organisation* 54.

BENERÍA, LOURDES (1979) 'Reproduction, production and the sexual division of labour', *Cambridge Journal of Economics* 3.

BEVAN, D., BIGSTEN, A., COLLIER, P., and GUNNING, J. W. (1988) 'Incomes in the United Republic of Tanzania during the "Nyerere experiment"', in W. van Ginneken (ed.), *Trends in Employment and Labour Incomes: Case Studies on Developing Countries*, Geneva: ILO.

BIEDELMAN, T. O. (1967) *The Matrilineal Peoples of Eastern Tanzania*, London: IAI.

BIENEFELD, M. A., and SABOT, R. H. (1972) *National Urban Mobility, Employment and Income Survey of Tanzania*, ii, Dar es Salaam: Ministry of Economic Affairs and Development Policy.

BINSWANGER, H., and MCINTIRE, J. (1987) 'Behavioral and material determinants of production relations in land abundant tropical agriculture', *Economic Development and Cultural Change* 36/1.

—— (1980) (eds.) *Rural Household Studies in Asia*, Singapore.

BLACKER, J. C. G. (1963) 'Population growth and natural increases in Tanganyika and Uganda' in J. Blacker and T. Smith (eds.), *Population Characteristics of the Commonwealth Countries of Tropical Africa.*

BLEDSOE, C. (1987) 'Side-stepping the post-partum sex taboo: Mende cultural perceptions of tinned milk in Sierra Leone', in E. van de Walle and J. Ebigola (eds.), *The Cultural Roots of African Fertility Regimes*, Ile-Ife and Philadelphia.

—— HILL, A., D'ALLESANDRO, U., and LANGEROCK, P. (1994) 'Constructing nutural fertility: the use of Western contraceptive technologies in rural Gambia, *Population and Development Review* 20/1.

BONGAARTS, JON, and POTTER, ROBERT (1983) *Fertility, Biology and Behaviour: An Analysis of the Proximate Determinants*, New York: Academic Press.

—— FRANK, ODILE, and LESTHAEGHE, RON (1984) 'The proximate determinants of fertility in sub-Saharan Africa', *Population and Development Review* 10/3.

—— BURCH, T. K., and WACHTER, K. W. (1987) (eds.) *Family Demography*, Oxford, Clarendon Press.

BRAIN, J. (1978) 'Symbolic rebirth: the *mwali* rite among the Luguru of Eastern Tanzania', *Africa* 48/2.

BRASS, W. (1975) *Methods for Estimating Fertility and Mortality from Limited and Defective Data*, Laboratory for Population Statistics, Carolina Population Center, University of North Carolina.

—— (1985) *Advances in Methods for Estimating Fertility and Mortality from Limited and Defective Data*, Centre for Population Studies, London School of Hygiene and Tropical Medicine.

—— (1987) 'The fertility transition in East Africa 1920–1970', Paper given at the Centre for Population Studies, London School of Hygiene and Tropical Medicine, 21 Jan. 1987.

—— (n.d.) 'Notes on fertility trends in Tanzania', Centre for Population Studies, LSHTM, mimeo.

BRYCESON, D. F. (1987) 'A century of food supply in Dar es Salaam' in J. Guyer (ed.), *Feeding African Cities*, Manchester: Manchester University Press.

—— (1988) 'Food insecurity and the social divison of labour in Tanzania 1919–1985', unpublished D.Phil thesis, University of Oxford.

BUJRA, JANET (1987) 'Men at work in the Tanzanian home: how did they ever learn?' Paper presented at Institute of Commonwealth Studies, London, Dec. 1987.

BURTON, RICHARD (1860) *The Lake Regions of Central Africa*, i, London.

CAIN, MEAD (1978) 'The household lifecycle and economic mobility in Bangladesh', *Population and Development Review* 4/3.

—— (1981) 'Risk and insurance: perspectives on fertility and agrarian change in India and Bangladesh', *Population and Development Review* 7/3.

—— (1983) 'Fertility as an adjustment to risk', *Population and Development Review* 4.

—— (1986) 'The consequences of reproductive failure: dependence, mobility and mortality among the elderly of rural South Asia', *Population Studies* 40/3.

CALDWELL, J. (1982) *Theory of Fertility Decline*, London: Academic Press.

—— and CALDWELL, P. (1981) 'The function of child spacing in traditional societies and the direction of change', in Page and Lesthaeghe (1981).

———— (1987) 'The cultural supports of high fertility in sub-Saharan Africa', *Population and Development Review* 13/3.

———— and QUIGGAN, P. (1989) 'The social context of AIDS in sub-Saharan Africa', *Population and Development Review* 15/2.

CAMPBELL, JOHN (1985) 'Neglect or disdain? The impact of two decades of urban policies toward the poor', Department of Sociology, University of Dar es Salaam, mimeo.

CAPLAN, A. P. (1975) *Choice and Constraint in a Swahili Community*, London: IAI.

—— (1976) 'Boy's circumcision and girl's puberty rites among the Swahili of Mafia Island, Tanzania', *Africa* 46.

—— (1981) 'Development policies in Tanzania: some implications for women', *Journal of Development Studies* 17/3.

—— (1982) 'Gender, ideology and modes of production on the coast of East Africa', *Paideuma* 28.

—— (1984) 'Cognatic descent, Islamic law and women's property on the East African Coast', in R. Hirschon (ed.), *Women and Property—Women as Property*, London, NY: Croom Helm/St Martin's.

CHATFIELD, W. R., SUTER, P. E. N., BREMNER, A. D., EDWARDS, E., and MCADAM, J. H. (1970), 'The investigation and management of infertility in East Africa', *East African Medical Journal* 47/4.

CHAYANOV, A. V. (1966) *The Theory of Peasant Economy*, Homewood, Ill.: Irwin.

CHESNAIS, J.-C. (1992) *The Demographic Transition*, Oxford: Clarendon Press.

CLAY, D., and J. VANDER HAAR (1993) 'Problems of intergenerational support and childbearing in the Third World', *Population Studies* 47.

CLELAND, JOHN (1985) 'Marital fertility decline in developing countries: theories and the evidence', in J. Cleland and J. Hobcraft (1985).

—— (1993) 'Equity, security and fertility: a reaction to Thomas', *Population Studies* 47/2.

—— and HOBCRAFT, J. (1985) (eds.) *Reproductive Change in Developing Countries*, Oxford: Oxford University Press.

—— and WILSON, CHRISTOPHER (1987) 'Demand theories of the fertility transition: an iconoclastic view', *Population Studies* 41/1.

COALE, A. J. (1968) 'Estimates of fertility and mortality in tropical Africa', in J. C. Caldwell and C. Okonjo (eds.), *The Population of Tropical Africa*, London: Longmans.

——(1973) 'The demographic transition re-considered', in *International Population Conference, Liège, 1973*, vol. I, Liège: IUSSP: 53–72.

——and DEMENY, P. (1983) *Regional Model Life-Tables and Stable Populations*, 2nd edn., Princeton: Princeton University Press.

——and WATKINS, S. C. (1986) (eds.) *The Decline of Fertility in Europe*, Princeton: Princeton University Press.

COHEN, G. (1978) *Karl Marx's Theory of History: A Defence*, Oxford: Clarendon Press.

COLEMAN, D., and SCHOFIELD, R. (1986) (eds.) *The State of Population Theory*, London: Macmillan.

COLLIER, P., RÀDWAN, S., and WANGWE, S. (1986) *Labour and Poverty in Tanzania*, Oxford: Clarendon Press.

COOK, ALISON (1974) *A Photo-interpretation Study of the Soils and Land-use Potential of the Lower Rufiji Basin*, Research Paper 3, Bureau of Resource Assessment and Land Use Planning, University of Dar es Salaam Dar es Salaam.

COONTZ, SIDNEY (1957) *Population Theories and the Economic Interpretation*, London: Routledge & Kegan Paul.

CORDELL, DENNIS, and GREGORY, JOEL (1980) 'Historical demography and demographic history in Africa: theoretical and methodological considerations', *Canadian Journal of African Studies* 14.

————and PICHÉ, VICTOR (1987) 'African historical demography: The search for a theoretical framework', in D. Cordell and J. Gregory (eds.), *African Population and Capitalism: Historical Perspectives*, Boulder, Colo.: Westview.

COULSON, ANDREW (1978) 'Agricultural policies in mainland Tanzania', *Review of African Political Economy* 10.

——(1982) *Tanzania: A Political Economy*, Oxford: Clarendon.

CROSS-UPCOTT, A. R. W. (1956) 'Social structure of the Ki-Ngindo speaking peoples', Unpublished PhD. thesis, University of Cape Town.

CULWICK, A. T., CULWICK, G. M. (1938/9) 'A study of population in Ulanga, Tanganyika Territory', *Sociological Review* 30/31.

DAVIS, K. (1963) 'The theory of change and response in modern demographic history' *Population Index* 29: 345–66.

DE JONGE, K., and STERKENBURG, J. (1973) 'The Rungwe survey', in Egerö and Henin (1973).

DETRAY, DENNIS (1976) 'Population growth and educational policies: an economic perspective', in Ridker (1976).

DONHAM, DONALD (1981) 'Beyond the domestic mode of production', *Man* 16/4.

EDHOLM, FELICITY, HARRIS, OLIVIA, and YOUNG, KATE (1977) 'Conceptualising women', *Critique of Anthropology* 9/10.

EGERÖ, B., and HENIN, R. A. (1973) (eds.) *The Population of Tanzania: An*

Analysis of the 1967 Population Census (Census vol. 6), Bureau of Resource Assessment and Land Use Planning, University of Dar es Salaam/Bureau of Statistics, Dar es Salaam.

ELLIS, FRANK (1980) 'A preliminary analysis of the decline in Tanzanian cashew nut production', Research Paper 79.1, Economic Research Bureau, University of Dar es Salaam.

EVANS, A. (1991) 'Gender issues in rural household economics', *IDS Bulletin*, 22/1: 51–9.

FEENEY, G. (1988) 'The use of parity progression models in evaluating family planning programmes', in *Proceedings of the African Population Conference, Dakar 1988* vol. 3, Liège: IUSSP.

FETTER, B. (1990) (ed.) *Demography from Scanty Evidence: Central Africa in the Colonial Period*, Boulder, Colo.: Lynne Rienner.

FOLBRE, N. (1986) 'Hearts and spades: paradigms of household economics', *World Development* 14/2.

FRANK, ODILE (1983) 'Infertility in sub-Saharan Africa: estimates and implications', *Population and Development Review* 9/1.

—— (1987) 'The demand for fertility control in sub-Saharan Africa', *Studies in Family Planning* 18/4.

FREEMAN-GRENVILLE, G. S. P. (1965) *The French at Kilwa Island*, Oxford: Oxford University Press.

GEIGER, SUSAN (1987) 'Women in nationalist struggle: TANU activists in Dar es Salaam', *International Journal of African Historical Studies* 20/1.

GIMENEZ, MARTHA (1977) 'Population and capitalism', *Latin American Perspectives* 4/4.

GLASSMAN, J. (1986) 'The roots of social rebellion in Pangani 1850–1888', Research Seminar Paper, Department of History, University of Dar es Salaam.

GLICK, P. C. (1947) 'The family cycle', *American Sociological Review* 12/2.

GOODY, ESTHER (1982) *Parenthood and Social Reproduction: Fostering and Occupational Roles in West Africa*, Cambridge: Cambridge University Press.

GOULBOURNE, H. (1978) 'Some aspects of ideological functions in the development of the post-colonial state in Tanzania', *Utafiti* 3/2.

GRAY, R. (1976) *Cambridge History of Africa*, iv, London: Cambridge University Press.

GREENHALGH, S. (1990) 'Towards a political economy of fertility: anthropological contributions', *Population and Development Review* 16/1.

GRILLICHES, Z. (1974) 'Comment' in Schultz (1976).

GUYER, JANE (1981) 'Household and community in African studies' *African Studies Review* 24/2–3.

GWASSA, G. C. K. (1972) 'Kinjikitile and the ideology of MajiMaji', in T. O. Ranger and I. N. Kimambo (eds.), *The Historical Study of African Religion*, London: Heinemann Educational.

—— and ILIFFE, J. (1967) (eds.) *Records of the MajiMaji Rising*, P. 1, Historical Association of Tanzania Paper 5, Dar es Salaam.

HAJNAL, JOHN (1953) 'Age at marriage and proportions marrying', *Population Studies* 7/2.

Handbook of German East Africa (1916) London.

HAMMEL, E. A. (1990) 'A theory of culture for demography', *Population and Development Review* 16/3.

HARRIS, OLIVIA, and YOUNG, KATE (1981) 'Engendered structures: some problems in the analysis of reproduction' in J. Kahn and J. Llobera (eds.) *The Anthropology of Pre-Capitalist Societies* London: Macmillan.

HARRISON, MARK (1982) 'Chayanov's theory of peasant economy', in J. Harriss (ed.), *Rural Development*, London: Hutchinson.

HART, G. (1980) 'Patterns of household labour allocation in a Javanese village', in Binswanger *et al.* (1980).

HARTWIG, GERALD (1979) 'Demographic considerations in East Africa during the 19th C', *International Journal of African Historical Studies* 12/4.

HAVNEVIK, KJELL (1983) *Analysis of Rural Production and Incomes, Rufiji District, Tanzania*, Research Paper 3, Institute of Resource Assessment, University of Dar es Salaam.

HILL, P. (1974) 'Big houses in Kano Emirate', *Africa* 44/2.

HO, THERESA J. (1979) 'Time costs of childrearing in the rural Philippines', *Population and Development Review* 5/4.

HÖHN, CHARLOTTE (1987) 'The family life cycle: needed extensions of the concept', in Bongaarts *et al.* (1987).

HULL, T. (1980) Comment on Nag, White, and Peet, in Binswanger *et al.* (1980).

HUNT, DIANA (1979) 'Chayanov's model of peasant household resource allocation', *Journal of Peasant Studies* 6/3.

HYDEN, G. (1980) *Beyond Ujamaa in Tanzania*, London: Heinemann.

ILIFFE, JOHN (1967) 'The organisation of the MajiMaji rebellion', *Journal of African History* 8/3.

—— (1969) *Tanganyika under German Rule*, Cambridge: Cambridge University Press.

—— (1970) 'A history of the dock workers of Dar es Salaam' *Tanzania Notes and Records* 71.

—— (1979) *A Modern History of Tanganyika*, Cambridge: Cambridge University Press.

KJEKSHUS, HELGE (1977) *Ecology Control and Economic Development in East African History: The Case of Tanganyika 1850–1950*, London: Heinemann.

KNAPPERT, JAN (1970) 'Social and moral concepts in Swahili Islamic literature' *Africa* 40/2.

KNODEL, J., and VAN DE WALLE, E. (1979) 'Lessons from the past: policy implications of istorical fertility studies', *Population and Development Review* 5/2.

KOPONEN, JUHANI (1986) 'Population growth in historical perspective: the key role of changing fertility', in J. Boesen (ed.), *Tanzania: Crisis and Struggle for Survival*, Uppsala: Scandinavian Institute of African Studies.

KREAGER, PHILLIP (1986) 'Demographic regimes as cultural systems', in Coleman and Schofield (1986).

KUCZYNSKI, R. R. (1949) *Demographic Survey of the British Colonial Empire, ii*, London: Oxford University Press.

KUZNETS, P. (1988) 'An East Asian model of economic development: Japan, Taiwan and South Korea', *Economic Development and Cultural Change* 37.

Lancet (1983) 'Malaria in Pregnancy', vol. 2, no. 8341 (9 July).

LANDBERG, PAMELA (1986) 'Widows and divorced women in Swahili society', in B. Potash (ed.), *Widows in Afircan Society* Stanford, Calif.: Stanford University Press.

LENIN, V. (1972) 'The differentiation of the peasantry', in J. Harriss (ed.), *Rural Development*, London: Hutchinson.

LERIDON, H., and MENKEN, J. (1979) (eds.) *Natural Fertility* Liège: IUSSP/Ordina.

LESLIE, J. A. (1963) *A Sociological Survey of Dar es Salaam*, Oxford: Oxford University Press.

LESTHAEGHE, R. (1980) 'On the social control of reproduction', *Population and Development Review* 6/4.

—— (1986) 'On sub-Saharan African systems of reproduction' in Coleman and Schofield (1986).

—— (1989*a*) (ed). *Reproduction and Social Organisation in Sub-Saharan Africa*, Berkeley and Los Angeles: University of Calfornia Press.

—— (1989*b*) 'Production and reproduction in Sub-Saharan Africa: an overview of organising principles', in Lesthaeghe (1989*a*).

—— and EELENS, F. (1989) 'The components of sub-Saharan reproductive regimes and their social and cultural components', in Lesthaeghe (1989*a*).

—— OHADIKE, P. O., KOCHER, J., and PAGE, H. (1981) 'Child spacing and fertility in sub-Saharan Africa: an overview of issues', in Page and Lesthaeghe (1981).

—— KAUFMANN, G., and MEEKERS, D. (1989) 'The nuptuality regimes in Sub-Saharan Africa', in Lesthaeghe (1989*a*).

LÉVI-STRAUSS, CLAUDE (1963) *Structural Anthropology*, Harmondsworth: Penguin.

LIENHARDT, PETER (1968) *Swifa ya Nguvumali: The Medicine Man*, Oxford: Oxford University Press.

LOCKWOOD, M. (1989*a*) 'The economics of fertility and the infertility of economics: theory and demographic reality in Africa', Working Paper 12, Centro Studi Luca d'Agliano, University of Turin/Queen Elizabeth House, Oxford University.

—— (1989*b*) 'Fertility and labour in Rufiji District, Tanzania', unpublished D.Phil thesis, University of Oxford.

—— (1992) 'Facts or fictions? Fieldwork relationships and the nature of data', in S. Devereux and J. Hoddinott (eds.) *Fieldwork in Developing Countries*, London, Harvester.

—— (1995) 'Structure and behavior in the social demography of sub-Saharan Africa', *Population and Development Review* 21/1.

—— (1996) 'Contrast and continuity in the African fertility transition: a cultural hypothesis', Research Paper 28, Geography Laboratory, University of Sussex.

Low, A. (1986) *Agricultural Development in Southern Africa: Farm Household Theory and the Food Crisis*, London: James Currey.

McNicoll, G. (1978) 'Population and development: outline for a structuralist approach', in Hawthorn (ed.), *Population and Development*, London: Frank Cass.

—— (1980) 'Institutional determinants of fertility change' *Population and Development Review* 6/3.

MajiMaji Research Project Collected Papers, Dar es Salaam.

Mamdani, Mahmood (1987) 'Extreme but not exceptional: towards an analysis of the agrarian question in Uganda', *Journal of Peasant Studies* 14/2.

Maro, P. (1974) 'Population and land resources in northern Tanzania: the dynamics of change 1920–1970', PhD thesis, University of Minnesota.

Marsland, H. (1938) 'Mlau cultivation in the Rufiji valley', *Tanzania Notes and Records* 5.

Martin, C. J. (1953) 'Some estimates of the general age distribution, fertility and rate of natural increase of the African population of British East Africa', *Population Studies* 7/2.

Marx, K. (1970) *Capital*, i, London: Lawrence & Wishart.

Mascarenhas, A. (1970) 'The Port of Dar es Salaam', *Tanzania Notes and Records* 71.

Mdemu, Chotigunga C. (1984) 'Nuptiality and fertility differences between migrants and non-migrants: A case study of Dar es Salaam city, Tanzania', unpublished thesis, Cairo Demographic Centre.

Meillassoux, Claude (1981) *Maidens, Meal and Money: Capitalism and the Domestic Community*, Cambridge: Cambridge University Press.

—— (1983) 'The economic bases of demographic reproduction: from the domestic mode of production to wage-earning', *Journal of Peasant Studies* 11/1.

Moore, H. (1988) *Feminism and Anthropology*, London: Polity.

Mueller, Eva (1976) 'The economic value of children in peasant agriculture', in Ridker (1976).

Nag, M., White, B., and Peet, R. C. (1980) 'An anthropological approach to the study of the economic value of children in Java and Nepal', in Binswanger *et al.* (1980).

Nelson, Nici (1987) 'Rural-urban child fostering in Kenya', in J. Eades (ed.) *Migrants, Workers and the Social Order*, London: Tavistock.

Nerlove, M. (1974) 'Toward a new theory of population and economic growth', in Schultz (1974).

Ngallaba, S. A. M. (1972) 'Fertility differentials in Tanzania with special reference to four Regions', MA thesis, University of Dar es Salaam.

Notestein, Frank (1945) 'Population: the long view', in T. W. Schultz (ed.), *Food for the World*, Chicago.

NUGENT, J. (1985) 'The old-age security motive for fertility', *Population and Development Review* 11/1.

NYERERE, JULIUS K. (1968) *Ujamaa—Essays on Socialism*, Dar es Salaam: Oxford University Press.

O'CONNOR, A. (1988) 'The rate of urbanisation in Tanzania in the 1970s', in M. Hodd (ed.), *Tanzania After Nyerere*, London: Pinter.

OLIVER, ROLAND (1977) *Cambridge History of Africa*, iii, London: Cambridge University Press.

ORDE-BROWNE, G. St. J. (1946) *Labour Conditons in East Africa*, London.

ORUBULOYE, O. (1981) 'Child spacing among rural Yoruba women', in Page and Lesthaeghe (1981).

PAGE, H. (1989) 'Childrearing versus childbearing: co-residence of mother and child in sub-Saharan Africa', in Lesthaeghe (1989*a*).

—— and LESTHAEGHE, RON (1981) (eds.) *Child Spacing in Tropical Africa: Traditions and Change*, London: Academic Press.

PAHL, R. (1984) *Divisions of Labour*, Oxford: Blackwell.

PATTERSON, K. D. (1981) 'The demographic impact of the 1918–19 influenza pandemic in sub-Saharan Africa: a preliminary assessment', in *African Historical Demography*, ii, Centre for African Studies, University of Edinburgh.

PAYER, C. (1983) 'Tanzania and the World Bank', *Third World Quarterly* 5/4.

PEARCE, RALPH (1986) 'Childlessness in Tanzania', unpublished MSc thesis, London School of Economics.

PEBLEY, A., and MBUGUA, W. (1989) 'Polygyny and fertility in sub-Saharan Africa', in Lesthaeghe (1989*a*).

POLGAR, STEPHEN (1972) 'Population history and population policies in an anthropological perspective', *Current Anthropology* 13/2.

POUWELS, R. (1987) *Horn and Crescent*, Cambridge: Cambridge University Press.

PRINS, A. H. J. (1967) *The Swahili-Speaking Peoples of Zanzibar and the East African Coast*, London: IAI.

RAHMAN, A. (1988) *Peasants and Classes*, London: Zed Press.

RANDALL, S., and WINTER, M. (1985) 'The reluctant spouse and the illegitimate slave', in A. Hill (ed.), *Population, Health and Nutrition in the Sahel*, London: Routleoge & Kegan Paul.

RIDKER, R. G. (1976) (ed.) *Population and Development*, Baltimore: Johns Hopkins University Press.

RIMMER, M. (1992) Unpublished D. Phil thesis, Cambridge University.

ROBERTS, D. S., and TANNER, R. E. S. (1959) 'A demographic study in an area of low fertility in north east Tanganyika', *Population Studies* 13/1.

ROBINSON, W. (1992) 'Kenya enters the fertility transition', *Population Studies* 46/3.

RODNEY, WALTER (1983) 'Migrant labour and the colonial economy', in W. Rodney, K. Tambila and L. Sago (eds.), *Migrant Labour in Tanzania during the Colonial Period*, Hamburg.

RUKONGE, A. D. (1985) 'The role of UMATI in child spacing in Tanzania' Dar es Salaam: UMATI, mimeo.

SABOT, R. (1979) *Economic Development and Urban Migration: Tanzania 1900–1971*, Oxford: Clarendon Press.

SAUCIER, J.-F. (1972) 'Correlates of the long post-partum taboo: a cross cultural study', *Current Anthropology* 13/2.

SAVILE, A. H. (1945) 'A study of recent alterations in the flood regime of three Tanganyikan rivers', *East African Agricultural Journal* 11.

SCHACHT, J. (1965) 'Notes on Islam in East Africa', *Studia Islamica* 23.

SCHOENMAECKERS, R., SHAH, I. H., LESTHAEGHE, R., and TAMBASHE, O. (1981) 'The child spacing tradition and the post-partum taboo in tropical Africa: anthropological evidence' in Page and Lesthaeghe (1981).

SCHULTZ, T. P. (1976) *The Economics of Population*, Reading, Mass.

SCHULTZ, T. W. (1974) (ed.) *Economics of the Family*, Chicago: Chicago University Press.

SEMBWAJE, I., S. L. (1984) 'The status of knowledge on mortality in Tanzania', *Utafiti* 6/2.

SEN, AMARTYA K. (1985) 'Women, technology and sexual divisions', *Trade and Development* 6.

SHANIN, T. (1987) (ed.) *Peasants and Peasant Societies*, Oxford: Blackwell.

SHANN, N. (1970) 'The educational development of the Chagga tribe' *Overseas Education* 26.

SHAPIRO, D. (1990) 'Farm size, household size and composition, and women's contribution to agricultural production: evidence from Zaire', *Journal of Development Studies* 27/1.

SHERIFF, A. (1987) *Slaves, Spices and Ivory in Zanzibar*, London: James Currey.

SHIVJI, I. (1986) *Law, the State and the Working Classes in Tanzania*, London: Heinemann.

SINGH, I., SQUIRE, L., and STRAUSS, J. (1986) *Agricultural Household Models: Extensions, Applications and Policy*, Johns Hophins University Press.

SMITH, R. (1981) 'Fertility, economy and household formation in England over three centuries', *Population and Development Review* 7/4.

SMITH, S., and SENDER, J. (1990) *Poverty, Class and Gender in Tanzania*, London: Routledge.

STANDING, H., and KÏSEKKA, M. (1989) *Sexual Behaviour in Sub-Saharan Africa: A Review and Annotated Bibliography*, London: Overseas Development Administration

STONE, J. (1990) 'Recollections of the annual population count in late precolonial Zambia', in Fetter (1990).

STROBEL, M. (1979) *Muslim Women in Mombasa 1890–1975*, New Haven: Yale University Press.

SUTTON, J. E. G. (1970) 'Dar es Salaam: a sketch of a hundred years', *Tanzania Notes and Records* 71.

SWANTZ, MARJA-LIISA (1970) *Ritual and Symbol in Transitional Zaramo Society*, Uppsala: C. W. K. Gleerup.

—— (1985) *Women in Development—A Creative Role Denied?*, London: Hurst/St Martins.

TAMBILA, K. (1983) 'A plantation labour magnet: the Tanga case', in W. Rodney, K. Tambila and L. Sago (eds.), *Migrant Labour in Tanzania during the Colonial Period*, Hamburg.

TANGANYIKA (1930–57) *A Digest of Appeals from Local Courts*, i–iv.

TANNER, R. E. S. (1962) 'The relationships between the sexes in a coastal Islamic society: Pangani District, Tanzania', *African Studies* 21/2.

TELFORD, A. (1929) *Report on the Development of the Rufiji and Kilombero Valleys*, London: Crown Aqents.

THOMAS, N. (1991) 'Land, fertility, and the population estalishment', *Population Studies* 45/3.

—— (1993) 'Economic security, culture and fertility: a reply to Cleland', *Population Studies* 47/2.

TITMUSS, RICHARD (1964) (ed.) *The Health Services of Tanganyika*, London: Pitman.

TOULMIN, C. (1992) *Cattle, Women and Wells*, Oxford, Clarendon Press.

TRIMINGHAM, J. S. (1964) *Islam in East Africa*, Cambridge: Cambridge University Press.

TURNER, V. (1967) *The Forest of Symbols* Ithaca, NY: Cornell University Press.

TUROK, B. (1975) 'The problem of agency in Tanzania's rural development: the Rufiji ujamaa scheme', in L. Cliffe *et al.* (eds.), *Rural Co-operation in Tanzania*, Dar es Salaam: Tanzania Publishing House.

TURSHEN, M. (1984) *The Political Ecology of Disease in Tanzania*, New Brunswick, NJ: Rutgers University Press.

UNITED NATIONS (1983) *Manual X: Indirect Techniques for Demographic Estimation*, New York.

—— (1992) *Child Mortality Since the 1960s*, New York.

United Republic of Tanzania (1973) *National Demographic Survey*, Bureau of Statistics.

VAN DE WALLE, E. (1992) 'Fertility transition, conscious choice and numeracy', *Demography* 29/4.

VAN HEKKEN, W., and VAN VELSEN, T. (1972) *Land Scarcity and Rural Inequality in Tanzania*, New York: Humanities Press.

VAUGHAN, M. (1991) *Curing Their Ills*, London: Polity.

VLASSOFF, C. (1990) 'The value of sons in an Indian village: how widows see it', *Population Studies* 44.

VOCK, JANE (1988) 'Demographic theories and women's reproductive labour', in S. Stichter and J. Papert (eds.), *Patriarchy and Class: African Women in the Home and the Workforce*, Boulder, Colo.: Westview Press.

VUORELLA, ULLA (1986) 'Relations of production among the matrilineal Kwere' Research Seminar Paper, History Dept., University of Dar es Salaam.

—— (1987) *The Women's Question and the Modes of Human Reproduction: An Analysis of a Tanzanian Village*, Finnish Society for Development Studies/Finnish Anthropological Society, Helsinki.

WATKINS, S. C., and MENKEN, J. (1985) 'Famines in historical perspective' *Population and Development Review* 11/4.

WEMBAH-RASHID, G. (1975) *The Ethno-History of the Matrilineal Peoples in South-East Tanzania, Acta Ethnologica et Linguistica* 32.

WESTERLUND, D. (1980) *Ujamaa na Dini: A Study of Some Aspects of Society and Religion in Tanzania 1961–1977*, Stockholm: Stockholm Studies in Comparative Religion, 18.

WHITEHEAD, A. (1981) '"I'm hungry, mum": the politics of domestic budgeting', in K. Young *et al.* (eds.), *Of Marriage and the Market*, London: CSE.

—— (1984) 'Beyond the household? Gender and kinship-based resource allocation in a Ghanaian domestic economy', Paper given at a conference on Conceptualising the Household, Harvard University.

—— (1990) 'Rural women in food production in sub-Saharan Africa', in J. Dreze and A. K. Sen (eds.), *The Political Economy of Hunger*, i, Oxford: Oxford University Press.

WILLIS, ROBERT J. (1973) 'A new approach to the economic theory of fertility' *Journal of Political Economy* 81/2.

—— (1982) 'The direction of intergenerational transfers and demographic transition: the Caldwell hypothesis re-examined', *Population and Development-Review* 8 (Supp. 82).

World Bank (1977) *Tanzania Basic Country Report: Annex III*, Washington, DC.

WRIGLEY, E. A., and SCHOFIELD, Roger (1981) *The Population History of England 1541–1871: A Reconstruction*, London: Edward Arnold.

YANAGISAKO, SYLVIA (1979) 'Family and household: the analysis of domestic groups', *Annual Review of Anthropology* 8.

YOSHIDA, M. (1974) *Agricultural Survey of the Lower Rufiji Plain*, unpublished MS.

Index

abortion 51, 54–5
abstinence, sexual 45, 46–8, 67–8, 92–4
adultery 89–90
age reporting 114
agricultural cycle 22, 86–7, 117–20
agricultural investment 71
amenorrhoea, post-partum 47–8
  see also breastfeeding; lactation
anaemia 50
Arusha Declaration 127

Bambara 18–19
Bangladesh 16, 153
birth intervals 38, 47–8, 51–2, 54–5, 92–4, 183
birth order 50
birth rate seasonality 49–50, 94
Bongaarts and Potter index 44, 48–9, 56–7
breastfeeding 4, 67, 92
  see also lactation; amenorrhoea, post-partum
brewing 119, 140, 149
bridewealth 96

capitalism 14–16
cash crops 119
  see also under specific crops
cashew nuts 133–6, 140
cassava 117–18, 163
censuses 28–30, 31–40
Chayanov, A. V. 101–9, 154–5, 168–9
child/adult ratio 27
childcare 115, 175–7
children 145–8
  benefits of 4–6, 14
  costs of 12
  demand for 4, 12
  and work 118, 175–7
Cleland, John 16–17
clothing 124
co-operation 102, 125, 163–8
coconuts 133–6
colonial administration 64, 79–80
  see also law
colonial period 23–4, 69–74
commodity prices 71, 81–5
contraception 3–4, 51–2, 54
contraceptive pill 52, 56
cosmology 66–8, 92
cotton 65–6, 88
crafts 119, 140
crop cultivation 81–5
  see also under specific crops

data collection 112–16
debt 72–3
decision making 11, 101
demographic transition 11, 14, 184–5
demography 101
  historical 23–4
dependency burden 168–70
dependency ratio 102, 153–5
divorce 46, 48, 87, 89–90, 148–9
  see also marital instability
domestic conflict 86, 88–9, 92–4, 125–6, 143–4, 177–8, 181
domestic violence 89

economic diversification 81–5, 165
economic mobility 102–4
education 78, 111–12
elderly 5, 14, 149
epidemics 24, 26–7
ethnic identity 59–60, 74–5

famine 23–7, 29, 72
fecundity 146
fertility 3–4, 35–41, 97, 183
  decline 16–19
  economic models 4–6, 11–12
  natural 5, 44–5, 48
  proximate determinants of 3–4, 17, 44–57
fieldwork 112–16
floods 20–2, 26
fostering 147–8

game reserves 71–2
gender relations 63–8, 87–8, 108–9
girls 66, 146, 174
Great Depression 28, 71

Hausa 18–19

health services 28
household 142–4
  composition 101–2, 152–5, 159–62, 164–5
    sex and age 108–9, 142, 170–2, 180
  economic activity 139–41, 165–72
  economy 12–16, 86, 101–7
  extension of 105, 160–2
  female headed 107, 138–9, 144, 148–9, 151, 154–5, 170
  formation and fission 149–53
  joint 150
  labour allocation 102–3, 164
  life cycle of 106–7, 142, 144–55
  and reproduction 142, 183
  size 105
  structure 107, 155, 164–8
  time allocation 113–16, 139–41, 173–4
  wealth 105, 132–41, 144, 160–1

illegitimacy 146–7
Indirect Rule 79–80
inequality 132–6
informal sector 78–9
intergenerational relations 96, 149
intergenerational transfers 13–14
Islam 20, 68, 69, 74–5, 87, 89–90, 92–3
  Sufism 75, 96
Islamization 87, 89

Jumbes 79–80

Kenya 20
kinship system 18, 59–63, 136, 148, 156
Koenigsberg 21

labour:
  demand 15
  domestic 180
  force 15, 77
  market 127–9
  relations 73–4
  supply 73, 102–4
  wage 102, 104, 127
lactation 45, 48, 93–4
  see also breastfeeding; amenorrhoea, post-partum
land acquisition 117
land allocation 128
land availability 104–6
land ownership 128–9, 132–3
law:
  colonial 89, 97
  Islamic, *see* sharia

Lenin, V. 102–7
Lesthaeghe, R. 44–5
lineage 61–3, 95, 111
lineage authority 79–80, 96, 128
Liverpool Uganda Company 129
living standards 84–5

MajiMaji war 64–6, 92
malaria 27, 45, 49–50
marital instability 46, 48, 53–4, 86–7, 148–9, 155–9
  see also divorce
marital status 54, 158, 172–4
marriage 58, 89, 183
  age at 19, 46, 52–4
  arranged 147
  child 147
  patterns 18–19, 58–63, 94–7
  payments 96
  and politics 60–3
Marxism 14–15
matriliny 18, 59–60
Meillassoux, Claude 1–3
men and work 90–2, 179–80
menarche 46, 145–6
merchants 70, 72, 130
migrants 59, 114
  education 78
  labour 129
  rural–urban 30–1, 75–9, 137
  sex ratio 30–1
modernization theory 11
Mohammed, Bibi Titi 75
mortality 23–8, 31–2
  child 33–5, 41
  infant 31–5, 41
  intrauterine 44–5, 47

National Demographic Survey 33–4, 37
new home economics 12–13
Nigeria 6, 18
nuclear family 152–3, 160–2

parity progression ratio 37–41
patriliny 60–3, 148
plantations 70, 73, 76
political organization 79–80
polygyny 46, 58, 97, 159–60
population:
  decline 24–8
  density 128
  growth 28–30, 42–3
  structure 28

pregnancy 92, 196–7
prices:
 crops 81–5
 food 77
Princeton European Fertility Project 11, 16, 23
property, personal 124–5, 136–7
puberty rites 46, 66–7, 145–7

questionnaires 112

rainfall 21–2, 129
relations of production 15–16
religious syncretism 89
reproduction 1–3, 183–5
rice 88–90, 91–2, 118–19, 165
 see also women and rice
rinderpest 26
risk 14
ritual 64
 see also cosmology; puberty rites
Rufiji (Tanzania):
 climate 21–2
 colonial history 69–74
 ecology 19–22
 economic history 69–74
 historical demography 23–43, 59–68
rural development policy 80–1, 111
rural economy 101, 117
Russia 101–2

sampling 113
seasonality, *see* agricultural cycle; birth rate seasonality; sexual division of labour, seasonal
settlement patterns 62, 80–1
sexual division of labour 65–6, 108–9, 117, 120–7, 130–1, 140, 169, 184
 seasonal 117–20
sexual intercourse 93–4
 frequency 50
sexuality 67
sharia 46, 89–90, 144, 148
smallpox 26
social change 4
soil type 21–2
sterility 19, 38, 45–8, 51, 54–5, 97, 155–8
stillbirth, *see* mortality, intrauterine
survey methods 112–16
swahili 74–5
syphilis 47

Tamasheq 18
Tanganyika African National Union (TANU) 75
Tanzania, *see* Rufiji
Tanzania Rural Development Bank 109
Tanzanian Demographic and Health Survey (TDHS) 34
taxation 46, 70, 87–8, 97, 124
time allocation, *see* household, time allocation
total fecundity rate 49
total fertility rate 17, 36, 49
trade 69–74, 130
 export, history of 25–6, 59, 72
transport 73
tree ownership 133–6

ujamaa villages 80, 95
Ukoo 128
UMATI (Tanzanian family planning association) 52
urbanization 30, 77

venereal disease 45–7
village organization 109–12
villagization 79–81, 94–5

wage levels 77
 urban 78–9
wealth accumulation 132
wealth flows 13
weaning 48, 68, 92
witchcraft 127
women:
 birth histories 114–15
 and education 95–6
 and Islam 75, 87, 89–90
 marriage histories 114
 and politics 75
 and property 144
 and rice 91–2, 127, 172–4, 180–1
 status 2
 and work 18–19, 87–92, 149, 172–8
working parties 126
World Bank 81
World Fertility Surveys 5, 16

Yoruba 6, 67

Zambia 28
Zaramo 67

The manufacturer's authorised representative in the EU for product safety is Oxford University Press España S.A. of el Parque Empresarial San Fernando de Henares, Avenida de Castilla, 2 – 28830 Madrid (www.oup.es/en or product.safety@oup.com). OUP España S.A. also acts as importer into Spain of products made by the manufacturer.

www.ingramcontent.com/pod-product-compliance
Lightning Source LLC
LaVergne TN
LVHW101502200926
848483LV00001B/197
* 9 7 8 0 1 9 8 2 8 7 5 4 4 *